Diets & Weight Loss

D1444439

by
Larry A. Richardson, M.D.

Banta Company
3300 Willow Spring Road
Harrisonburg, VA 22801
703.564.3900

About the Author

Larry A. Richardson, M.D. is a practicing Bariatrician and member of The American Society of Bariatric Physicians and The North American Association for the Study of Obesity. Dr. Richardson is Board Certified in Emergency Medicine and has a special interest in Preventative Medicine.

Notice of liability

The information in this book is distributed on an "As is" basis, without warranty. While every precaution has been taken in the preparation of this book, neither the author nor printer, shall have any liability to any person or entity with respect to any liability, loss, or damage caused or alleged to be caused directly or indirectly by the instructions, suggestions, and material contained in this book. It is the responsibility of each person to discuss material in this book with their own physician before beginning recommendations contained herein.

Trademarks

The majority of the contents of this book are based upon the *Sir Cadian Weight Management Program*. **Sir Cadian** and **Sir Cadian...It's About Time** are trademarks of Larry A. Richardson, M.D., P.A. Throughout this book trademarks of other entities are used. Rather than put a trademark symbol in every occurrence of a trademarked name, the author is using the names only in an editorial fashion and to the benefit of the trademark owner with no intention of infringement of the trademark.

What is *Sir Cadian?*

The *Sir Cadian* program is a comprehensive weight management program developed and supervised by Larry A. Richardson, M.D. It is based on the notion that ***circadian*** relates to *24 hour cycles* seen in many living organisms—with events tending to occur at the same time each day. Weight management is a **daily** event, based on our choices and activities. The *Sir Cadian* program also strives to encourage participants to consume the greatest quantities of foods at **times** early in the day as fat cells may have increased susceptibility to storing lipids during certain hours of the day. Hence, ***it's about time*** that someone came up with *sensible* weight management . We feel this is such a program.

Library of Congress Catalog Card Number: 93-93661
ISBN 0-9636840-1-9

0 9 8 7 6 5 4 3 2 1
Printed and bound in the United States of America

Larry A. Richardson, M.D., P.A.
2031 Humble Place Drive
Humble, Texas 77338
713.540.2422

Dedication

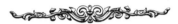

First, and foremost, this book is dedicated to my best friend and wife, Joan. She has been a true inspiration to me to keep going when the going got rough. In fact, this book would not have been possible without her relentless dedication to me and our family. Many a night she had to keep the home fires burning and help the children with their homework or run errands for them so dad could work on this book. Anyone helped by the material contained herein owes her a debt of gratitude also. She truly is the 'unsung hero' that helps to make my job easier.

This book is also dedicated to my pre-med advisor, Dr. Joyce Fan. It was her sing-song of 'al-DE-hyde' and other memory mnemonics which helped make organic chemistry bearable. She inspired me to look at complex things in a simple way. This ultimately paved the way to my intérest in medicine and a medical career. In that same spirit of simplicity, I have attempted to take a look at the complex issue of dieting and weight management and to simplify it wherever possible. My hope is that this book will encourage its readers to do small things consistently, rather than large things inconsistently. To good food and good health....It's About Time.

Contents

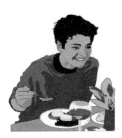
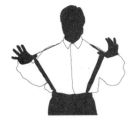

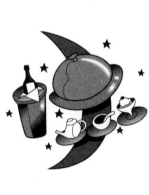

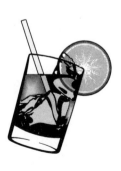

NOTICE

Before beginning this or any other medical or nutritional regimen, consult a nutrition-oriented physician to be sure it is medically appropriate for you.

The information in this book is not intended to replace medical advice. Any medical questions, general or specific, should be addressed to your physician.

NOTES:

Introduction

Most obesity programs and books have but one primary goal—weight loss. Previously it may have been acceptable to focus on a specific weight, but could such tunnel-vision be contributory to the ever increasing amounts of psychological and eating disorders we are experiencing in this country?

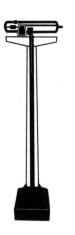

This book is not about what you *lose* but about what you *gain*. Through nutrition education, behavior modification, and counseling you can *gain* an understanding of what body weight actually is, how it's managed, and methods to help you control it for a lifetime. If you want to lose weight and keep it off, you must realize that you will never be able to return to your previous eating *habits*. You will learn about *balance*—balance in eating, activity, and expectations. You will see what can be accomplished with a healthy way of living and not just some short-lived method of losing.

Once you undertake changing your lifestyle, knowing where you have been becomes a map to plot your course for the future. One of the most difficult concepts to overcome is doing away with unrealistic goal weights. Some of the most knowledgeable experts in the field of obesity are now saying that it is *amount of body fat*, not total body weight, that is crucial and should be targeted for control in weight management.

Even *low weight* individuals can have excessive body fat. Some of it may be marbled throughout their muscle mass. Some may be hidden within the abdominal cavity, wrapped silently around organs, including the heart. In contrast, you may begin a healthy lifestyle, including becoming more active, and actually *gain weight* as you build muscle. Don't let normal physiological changes discourage you. They become less threatening when you understand what is really going on.

"This book is not about what you lose but about what you gain."

Accumulated fat is on our bodies for a multitude of reasons. The ways people try to remove the accumulation are even more numerous. However, truly safe ways are few, and the ways to keep it off are even fewer.

Just by acquiring this book, you have overcome two of the most difficult hurtles in the management of this problem. You have (1) recognized you have a problem, and (2) you have sought help for that problem.

The final step that must be taken is a *change in habits*, probably habits of a lifetime. That's the tough part, isn't it? Old habits helped you put on that fat. It will take new habits to lose it and keep it off. Did you have to go on a diet to put that fat on? Then why keep believing that it will take a *diet* to rid yourself of excessive fat?

Are you tired of setting yourself up for failure? Are you sick of the dieting rut? De-program and climb out of the rut today—right now! You will no longer have to diet! Diets imply a short-term commitment. You will eat [or learn to eat again] in a

"...make a commitment... to yourself..."

different light. A non-threatening, scientific, logical, and sensible approach to eating choices and food attitudes will be presented in these pages.

It will be up to you as to whether you will choose to follow the simple guidelines of this program. You are in control. *You must make a commitment*—not to a program, but to yourself—and that commitment is for changes in *lifestyle and food selection.*

Before we can begin to understand nutrition, we need to realize that the majority of those reading this book are *malnourished* . . . overweight, but malnourished. Ironic isn't it? Living in one of the greatest food-producing nations on earth and yet we are malnourished. Few of us would really consider *obesity* as a form of malnutrition, yet it is the most common type in the United States. It is a by-product of affluence and our increasingly sedentary lifestyles.

It is time we quit playing games and making jokes about our excess adiposity. Obesity is one of several major influences that contribute to *atherosclerotic vascular disease*, the leading cause of death in the United States. Other factors include inactivity, cigarette smoking, and high blood pressure.

Just being 5% overweight can shorten your life. Every extra pound adds extra miles of capillaries and blood vessels that your heart must work harder for. Excess body fat is associated with arthritis of weight-bearing joints, back problems, cancer, cardiovascular disease, menstrual and fertility difficulties, respiratory problems, stroke, and varicose veins.

Of those using various dieting methods, only about one in ten achieve and maintain their desired weight loss beyond one to five years after losing it initially. Don't let this be a source of discouragement, but instead let it serve to motivate you in the discipline, vigilance, and commitment you *must* have to achieve this worthwhile goal.

"...98% of the fats we eat go directly to our fat stores."

Safe weight loss has no shortcuts. It requires time and effort. Too many empty calories (usually supplied by dietary fats) cause oversupply for our nutritional needs. This in turn creates more fats. It has been said that ninety-eight percent of the fats we eat go directly to our fat stores. What a confirmation of the old saying, "You are what you eat!".

Don't let your good intentions get sidetracked when something comes along that looks easier. No book, potion, pill, chocolate shake, subliminal tape, exercise video or other single method can do as much for you as this simple program of getting back to the basics.

How long did it take you to put on your extra fat? Aren't a few weeks or months worth the trouble to take it off sensibly? Once the weight is lost, many successful maintainers have developed the knack of keeping lowfat foods high in appeal and low on boredom. This can be done through a host of options including lowfat recipes and trying spice, herb, and special seasoning combinations.

The fundamentals of this program need to be a *lifelong commitment*. Take one day at a time. Set short-term goals for the next few days or just the week ahead. Don't try to do all of the suggestions in this book in one great big chunk. Any job is easier when you break it down into smaller parts. The same is true of weight management. It's definitely easier to strive for moderation rather than total elimination of certain foods and habits. It also tends to make for more successful weight loss long term. Individuals who relapse on their weight tend to deny themselves enjoyable food while losing.

Decide here and now if loss of fat and weight reduction is what you *really* want. Some of you reading this may have been traumatized or sexually abused as a child and have built up an unconscious desire to be overweight as a defense mechanism to be *unattractive* to prevent further abuse. You may find certain advantages in remaining overweight, such as avoiding close, intimate relationships.

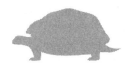

"Remember the story of the tortoise and the hare."

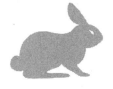

Physicians are finding ever increasing numbers of patients with excess weight problems that had early psychological and physical trauma. If you relate to this situation, get professional psychological help to work through some of these deep-seeded emotions—even before you continue with this or any program. To be successful, you must address the root of the problem. Even if things previously mentioned are not the root of your problem, you must recognize whether one part of you is resisting losing weight. If so, specifically identify what is causing the resistance and then make a deliberate choice as to what is truly your desire in regards to your weight.

Put determination into your efforts and nothing will be able to stop you. Remember the story of the tortoise and the hare. Jackrabbit starts may look wonderful, but it is steady, determined persistence that wins out. Weight management is no different.

If you feel you have a special medical problem that would prevent you from following some of the recommendations in this book, please discuss your concerns with your personal physician. While the guidelines in this book will help you during your weight management program, no set of rules or suggestions can promise everyone good health and lack of problems.

Many factors can govern your overall health. Personality may influence your risk factors, as can mental health. Heredity you can't change, but why not work on changing a poor environment, destructive lifestyle, or improper nutrient intake?

"You are no longer alone in your quest..."

You are no longer alone in your quest to see yourself thinner and healthier. The author of this book understands and cares. Join me now, through the remaining pages of this book, and incorporate its simplicity and truths into your life. You are again in control. You have been given a key. It is up to you which locks you will open with it.

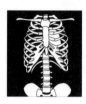

Maintain Healthy Weight

If you are too fat or too lean, your chance of developing health problems is increased. Being *too fat* is linked with high blood pressure, heart disease, stroke, diabetes, certain cancers, and other types of illness. Being *too thin* is a less common problem, but it is linked with osteoporosis in women and greater risk of early death in both women and men.

Whether your weight is *healthy* depends on how much of your total weight is fat, where in your body the fat is located, and whether you have weight-related medical problems or a family history of such problems.

What is a healthy weight for you? There is no totally accepted answer right now. Researchers are developing more precise ways to measure healthy weight and may have some recommendations for us in the near future. In the meantime, you can assess your weight this

TABLE 1

Weight ranges in pounds for various heights

Height	19 to 34 years old	35 years and over
5' 0"	97-128	108-138
5' 1"	101-132	111-143
5' 2"	104-137	115-148
5' 3"	107-141	119-152
5' 4"	111-146	122-157
5' 5"	114-150	126-162
5' 6"	118-155	130-167
5' 7"	121-160	134-172
5' 8"	125-164	138-178
5' 9"	129-169	142-183
5' 10"	132-174	146-188
5' 11"	136-179	151-194
6' 0"	140-184	155-199
6' 1"	144-189	159-205
6' 2"	148-195	164-210
6' 3"	152-200	168-216
6' 4"	156-205	173-222
6' 5"	160-211	177-228

(Height above without shoes. Weight without clothes.)

"Heredity plays a role in body size and shape..."

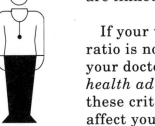

way: see if yours is a weight believed to be in the acceptable range for persons of your age and height, as shown in **Table 1**.

Weights *above* the range in table 1 are linked to increased risk to health. Weights *below* the range may be healthy; but are sometimes linked to health problems, especially if sudden weight loss occurs.

Next, consider your *body shape*. Excess weight in the *abdomen* is believed to be of greater health risk than that in the hips and thighs. To check your body shape, measure around your waist where it is smallest while you stand relaxed, not pulling in your stomach. Then, measure around your hips where they are largest. Divide the waist measurement by the hips measurement to get your *waist-to-hip ratio*. Ratios above 0.80 for women and 0.95 for men are linked to greater risk for several diseases.

If your weight is within the range in the table, if your waist-to-hip ratio is not high-risk, and if you have no medical problem for which your doctor recommends weight gain or loss, there appears to be *no health advantage to changing your weight*. If you do not meet all of these criteria, you may wish to discuss your weight and how it might affect your health with your doctor.

Heredity plays a significant role in body size and shape, as does exercise and what you eat. Some people can eat heartily and still not be too heavy. Others have difficulty achieving a good weight and shape even with dieting. You will find other tips and explanations for these and other aspects of weight management throughout the remainder of this book.

THE BOTTOM LINE

True overall health comes from mental, physical, and spiritual well being. Success in all of these areas comes from a balance of many factors. It is the extremes that generally get people into trouble. As a physician, I can address the first two aspects. Your minister or clergy should be able to give you guidance about the spiritual realm.

"True overall health comes from mental, physical, and spiritual well being."

If you are interested in learning more about spiritual matters, feel free to contact me at the address located in the front of this book (copyright page). I will be happy to send you further reading material that may help you learn more about this important aspect of yourself and your needs.

Quick Start

Knowing that there are those of you who desire to get maximum benefit with minimum reading and instructions, I will try to encapsulate the essence of this book in the next several paragraphs. For those desiring the bare minimum of instruction, this entire *Quick Start* section is dedicated. For the remainder of readers (hopefully a majority), the entire book is a resource of suggestions, tips, encouragement, and guidelines.

As for my recommendation, *I encourage everyone to thoroughly read through this book*, including sections covering risks and warnings, before undertaking a program of weight reduction and management. This book is not meant to be *all inclusive* of the multiple factors and risks governing weight reduction but merely a guide to some of the more common ones.

"...get a complete physical exam..."

You are also advised to get a complete physical examination, as well as discuss the advisability of weight reduction with your own family physician prior to beginning any weight reduction program. This program is a supplement to, not a replacement for, your family or personal health care provider. If you have a physical or hormonal problem, your physician's participation is essential.

It is generally accepted that obesity has many causes and that an individual is usually overweight due to interactions of several of these. Since there can be a multitude of contributing factors, it makes sense to approach weight loss and management from many angles. In fact, it is the multifactorial research studies that seem to have the best long-term weight maintenance success (calorie and fat monitoring, increased physical exercise, behavioral modification, training in relapse prevention techniques, continued contact via mail, phone, or in person, etc.).

Not everyone trying to lose weight needs to, and in some, it may actually be more harmful to attempt to do so. Weight cycling (gain-lose-gain) certainly has its own inherent set of problems. Be sure to read more about this elsewhere in this book.

Some people 20% or more over their ideal weight may be encouraged to reduce weight for health reasons depending upon their circumstances. Obesity is known to increase the risk of disease and death from certain medical problems. On the other hand, other diseases can aggravate the problems associated with obesity.

Current recommendations by some national advisory committees set a *goal of reducing weight by 10%* in moderately overweight individuals, which can improve health risks in some individuals. A steady loss of 1/2 to 1 pound a week until such goal is reached is generally considered safe, especially if not monitored by a physician. It also seems to be a level of loss that is realistic to maintain, based on multiple long-term studies.

Factors Correlated with Weight Loss:

1. Self-monitoring
2. Goal setting
3. Social support
4. Treatment length

The old *basic four food groups* and the recommended levels of intake for each group have been updated dramatically. The Department of Agriculture is promoting their food guide pyramid which gives different emphasis (weights) to different food groups. Today, eating should be more consistent than what you may have done to in the past—emphasizing more vegetables, fruits, whole grains, and complex carbohydrates.

Adequate dietary protein is important but debates rage over what constitutes proper levels and how much is actually needed. The proper level does vary during weight loss. Most authorities agree that it is *fat consumption* by Americans that is excessive and should be *reduced to 30% or less* of intake. Saturated fats seem to be the worse dietary fats.

Factors Correlated with Wt. Maintenance Long Term

1. Self-monitoring
2. Exercise
3. Continued monitoring by wt. monitoring providers

Average caloric intake for *low-calorie diets* seem to range from about 800 to 1200 calories. Most *very-low-calorie diets* consisting of 800 calories or less are not recommended outside of hospital and/or close physician monitoring situations. Dropping calories too low has been found to *reduce* basal metabolic rate and cause *excessive protein loss*. It also tends to lead to bingeing and 'diet failure'. Crash diets are to be avoided as they tend to lose almost as much muscle as fat, as well as reducing resting metabolic rate.

Vitamin and mineral supplements, including calcium, potassium, and other electrolytes are often recommended for low caloric diets. Fluid intake is equally essential, and recommended amounts are at least eight to ten (and more) 8-ounce glasses of fluid per day.

Exercise is important but emphasis seems to be shifting away from the necessity of aerobics three times or more a week towards just increasing activities of daily living (e.g. stand while talking on the telephone, taking stairs instead of elevators, etc.). "Just be more active than you ordinarily are" seems to be a theme being echoed over and over at obesity conferences.

Strenuous exercise, in combination with low calories, has been noted [in some studies] to actually *reduce overall metabolic rate*, rather than enhance it as was previously thought. No matter what other benefits it produces, it has *not* been shown to cause large weight reduction in obese individuals. The good news is that being just *a little* more physically fit can significantly reduce the risk of death in many overweight individuals.

In summary, the following factors are correlated with weight loss: self-monitoring (food diaries, periodic weighing), goal setting (realistic; not *ideal*), social support (significant others), and treatment length (generally more weight lost with longer treatment times). Factors associated with long-term weight maintenance include self-monitoring , exercise (both planned and daily physical activity increase), and continued contact with weight monitoring providers (physicians, dietitians, counselors, support groups, etc.).

Weight re-gain has been found to sometimes stem from binge (or emotional) eating, poor (negative) coping mechanisms, and situational or life stress. Some people find that by just controlling their binge eating, they can ultimately reduce their weight. Unrealistic weight goals can also be partially responsible for failure to maintain weight loss.

FUNDAMENTALS TO WEIGHT REDUCTION:

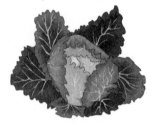

To eat less food:
- Have smaller portions of foods you wish to limit.
- Make small changes gradually.
- Consume higher bulk, more filling, and less caloric foods.
- Remove plate when finished to diminish nibbling.
- Place leftovers into garbage or refrigerator/freezer immediately.

To eat less high-fat items:
- Choose lower-fat foods or modify food to lowfat when possible.
- Eat more vegetables, whole grains, and fruits.
- Replace high-fat meat dishes with pasta, potatoes, and rice dishes.
- Eat high-fat foods on a limited basis.

To eat fewer empty calories:
- Substitute lower-calorie foods gradually.
- Reduce high sugar foods and sweets in general.
- Reduce intake of items with lots of highly refined sugars and/or flour.
- Consume fewer alcoholic beverages.

To lose weight appropriately:
- Do not induce vomiting or purge (can cause irregular heartbeats and death).
- Do not abuse laxatives (body may become dependent on them).
- Do not try to modify all eating habits in one day or one week.
- Make changes in areas that allow you to regain control over eating.
- Be aware of what and when you are putting things in your mouth.
- Target binge eating.

To adapt a proper mental attitude:
- Avoid restrictive dieting.
- Set realistic goal weights.
- Focus on health rather than appearance.
- Focus on self-esteem.

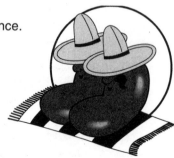

Program Directions

This book is loaded with tips, information, and guidelines that can help with weight management. In this section, we will try to look at a few highlights and list some generalities that you should attempt while on this program. Further explanations and tips for these guidelines can be found elsewhere in this book.

I feel my role is similar to that of a coach. This means I will give you tips to help you develop your full potential. This is in contrast to where I would function as a dictator, demanding that you do this or that and giving you menus and do's and don'ts written in stone.

"This program is not just another diet..."

In getting started, you need to realize the chronicity of the problem. For most, it's a lifetime vigilance. There will be times when you *fall off the wagon* or slip back into old, unhealthy habits or lifestyles. It's not that you will never falter, but you should learn to adapt and handle these times constructively. Therefore adopt an attitude of flexibility and creativity in your therapy. I hope that you will grasp this spirit to improve your quality of life. Maintenance of healthy eating and exercise habits becomes your therapeutic goal, rather than just some number on a scale.

The true measure of success comes when you adopt a healthy lifestyle. Put aside old ways and out-dated attitudes. What possible benefit could they be to you now? They will only keep you from being all that you can be—more motivated, more energetic, and more attractive. This program is not just another *diet* but is a back-to-the-basics way of eating and living which you can utilize for the rest of your life. "U" and your direct participation are the important part of any sUccess.

A good weight management program should address several areas—moderation, consistency, and avoiding craziness. It should stress these areas in the realm of sensible eating, regular exercise, behavior changes to control bingeing or over-eating, and should be both positive and motivational. *Moderation* can be accomplished by using several approaches to the same problem. In so doing, modest interventions can be used to achieve the desired results. Secondly, *consistency* means doing small things continually rather than large things occasionally. Stop looking for *quick fixes* and begin looking at the long-term picture.

"Avoiding extremes is good advice..."

The last topic, *avoiding craziness*, can be addressed by just avoiding the thousands of fad diets that come and go, setting realistic goals and weights, and not trying to overdo caloric restriction or attempt excessive exercise in an attempt to punish ourselves and make up for lost time. Avoiding extremes is good advice in life and certainly applies to weight management.

General Guidelines

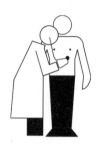

In the Beginning

- Before starting your weight management program, see your doctor for a medical checkup if you have not had one recently. Get your physician's approval for weight reduction if you have medical problems.
- Keep a diary of food and exercise. This is not something indefinite but has been shown to help people lose more weight and have a better chance at keeping it off. Recording makes you focus on habits and allows you to think about wiser choices. It also keeps you honest and helps overcome *calorie amnesia*.

"Keep a diary of food and exercise."

Know What Works

- Don't worry about the size of your plate, just the *calories* and *fats* you get from what is on your plate.
- If weight plateaus, resume your daily calorie journal.
- Even when stressed, tired, depressed, or bored, try to limit yourself to bulky, nutrient-filled foods and skip the high-fat ones. Nutrients feed your hunger. Empty calories feed your fat (e.g. sugars, refined flours, butters, creams, sauces, dressings, finger-foods, etc.).

Caloric Restriction

"There is no food that cannot occasionally be eaten..."

No more "never agains".

- There is no food that cannot occasionally be eaten (e.g. cake, chocolate, dessert, wine), but obviously we need to modify certain *quantities* and frequencies of various types of food.
- Do avoid fad diets which do nothing to change your long-term eating behavior. Eat at least three moderately-sized nutritional meals. Don't skip meals as you will be more likely to snack on high calorie foods.
- Allow yourself to eat *problem* foods in controlled settings, especially in front of other people. Set a limit and stick to it.

Abandon the *dieting* concept.

- Dieting is a very negative concept. Diets mean restrictions and since you didn't have to go on a diet to gain the extra weight, why must you go on one to lose it?
- Plan your own meals rather than just grabbing haphazardly whatever happens to be convenient. You are in charge of your life and no one should force you to eat or not eat something. Just adapt to eating *more* basic nutrients and *less* empty calories (possibly taste satisfying but certainly short-lived).
- Try to start out keeping a food diary. Think of it like a checkbook. It will allow you to track your eating behavior (and calories) to give you an idea of what is really going on in your eating habits.
- If you have been a chronic dieter, it may take 6-12 weeks to increase your metabolic rate by proper eating techniques. Begin by not skipping breakfast and try to space your food intake throughout the day.

"Choose lower-fat, lower-calorie foods."

Consume at least 900 calories daily.

- A *low-calorie* program of between 900-1100 calories daily sometimes works for select individuals. Long-term consumption of less than 800 calories puts you into a *very-low-calorie* program and increases potential risk. It therefore requires closer medical supervision due to increased potential of mood and electrolyte changes, depression, weakness, syncope, muscle loss, uncontrollable appetite, and decreased body metabolism. Even on 1000 calories some people stay hungry and eventually relapse to their old eating habits. A weight counselor can work with you on your optimum intake.
- A 1,200 or more calorie per day diet is called a *balanced deficit diet*. Such calorie intake is usually low enough to induce weight loss in most people. For some very large people, even 1,200 calories a day may be too low.
- Diabetics and other select patients may need additional calories. Check with your family physician.
- Choose lower-fat, lower-calorie foods. Eat more fruits, whole grains, and vegetables. Eat less high fat and high sugar items and consume less alcoholic beverages.
- Try to eat about 55-67% of your calories as complex carbohydrates (fruits, vegetables, starches), 15-20% protein (fish, poultry, meat, dairy), and <30% fat every day while attempting weight reduction. You should consume at least 1 gram of protein for every kilogram of ideal body weight. [This is the same as about 1/2 gram of protein intake per pound ideal weight.]
- Eat smaller portions of foods you need to limit and substitute lower-calorie foods gradually.
- Consume adequate amounts of fluids. Drink 8-12 glasses of fluid (preferably water) each day. Try having water 20 minutes before meals and with them also.

Consume calories early

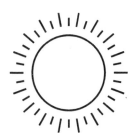

- Try to consume the majority of your calories early in the day. A goal could be to eat 3/4 of your daily total by 6 to 7 hours after awakening.
- Supper should consistently be your *lightest* calorie meal, not the heaviest. Circadian cycles within the body may make your fat cells more receptive to storing fats at certain times of the day compared to other times. Unfortunately, these times may be more in the evenings and early morning hours in overweight individuals.
- Many obese individuals typically skip breakfast and consume the majority of their calories from supper to bedtime. One reason some eat so much in the evening hours is that they have gone without nutrient intake most of the day and their body (and appetite) finally catches up with them.

Medications

What to Expect (if your physician has you on medication for weight control):

"Medications mainly deal with internal cues to eating."

- **Only take medication as prescribed. NEVER increase the dose or frequency on your own! It could be dangerous (even deadly).** This can be true of *any* prescription medication.
- While medication can assist you in losing weight, it is up to you to maintain your health through proper eating and not improper *dieting*.
- You can *eat through* any medication. No pill or potion will make you put down the dessert or chocolate bar. You must do so of your own free will. This puts you back in control.

•Medications mainly deal with internal cues to eating. You should help curb your appetite by feeding it bulky and filling nutrients and plenty of fluids. Habits must be changed if the weight loss is to be permanent.

• Controversy exists as to duration of medication use in treatment of obesity. However, some leading researchers are beginning to advocate long-term use of medications in weight therapy. They argue that hypertension and diabetes return when medications are stopped for those conditions. They see a double standard in the attitude that appetite suppressants should only be used for a few weeks, yet the weight loss is expected to be maintained without pharmacological help.

•If you are reducing calories on your own, you should probably take a multivitamin and mineral supplement.

Eating Guidelines

"Eat at set times and places."

Settings and Situations

•Eat slowly by planning enough time to eat, cutting food into smaller pieces, chewing slower, putting your fork down between bites, and perhaps taking a break during the meal.

•Eat at set times and places. Choose one place to eat and *only eat there*. Plan snacks, special occasions, and occasional desserts to overcome the feeling of deprivation.

•Don't eat while engaged in another activity, such as reading or watching TV. Concentrate on the *act* of eating.

•Today, most restaurants have diet drinks and low-calorie plates and single menu items. You won't be looked down upon for ordering these.

Suggestions

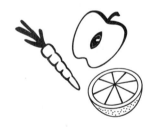

•Eating a high-fiber breakfast gives you a good start to the day and helps reduce high calorie snacking.

•Avoid fried foods, high-fat snacks and high-fat fast foods, and use minimal amounts of fat and oil. Trim fat from meat and skin from poultry. Utilize lowfat dairy products and low-calorie dressings and toppings. Use fat-free cooking methods whenever possible. Limit nuts. Modify everything to be lowfat when possible.

•Eat adequate fresh fruits, vegetables, and whole-grain products. Besides being healthier, they can also help with constipation.

•Desirable low-calorie snacks include apples, oranges, carrot sticks and other raw vegetables, and plain popcorn.

Social Situations

•When dining out, avoid fried and sauce-covered dishes as well as pastries, salad dressings, and desserts. Try water with lemon or mineral water as a beverage.

•Don't come to a meal *starved*. Have a piece of fruit, a small salad or some soup beforehand if needed.

•When people socialize, there tends to be lots of food and drink. In fact, many people think that the mark of a good host or hostess is getting guests to eat and drink as much as possible. Counter this with being honest with those with whom you will be socializing. Elicit their cooperation and they should realize you are not being antisocial, just health conscious. If they have any sensitivity, they will help you by not shoving food and drinks at you.

•No matter how much you plan, large gatherings tend to have at least one insensitive

"Exercise was not designed specifically to lose weight..."

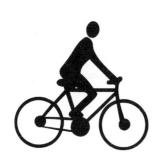

person who does their best to get you to eat and drink something (usually of their choosing). Sometimes the best way to deal with such a person is to be very direct and assertive. Saying you will have something 'later' may help.

Exercise

Expectations

- It takes a great deal of exercise to offset excessive calorie (and fat) intake.
- Exercise was not designed specifically to lose weight but it can help you to feel better. Lose the weight and consult your doctor regarding a proper pre-exercise evaluation. A stress test (treadmill) checks your heart during activity and is a wise precaution before undertaking a program of moderate exercise. It is recommended if (a) you are 45 or over, (b) you are between age 35-44 and have at least one risk factor for coronary artery disease (family history, smoking, high blood pressure or cholesterol, or obesity), or (c) have diabetes, hyperthyroidism, lung or cardiovascular disease (stress test may cause some risk so consult your physician first).

Basic Guidelines

- Begin slowly and work towards consistency and cardiovascular fitness.
- As a minimum, just increase activities of daily living (e.g. use the stairs, stand while talking on the phone, etc.). Keep moving as much as possible throughout the day. Don't expect this to substitute for an exercise regimen though.
- Base exercise on your preferences and try to participate in several types in order to have variety and alternatives.
- For those wishing to participate in aerobic exercise (after medically evaluated), a goal of 3 to 5 times a week of 30-45 minutes seems to be a reasonable standard.
- Maintenance exercise is quite important and has a high correlation with successfully maintaining weight long-term.

Behavior Modification

Basics

- The fundamentals of proper therapy are to help you consume less empty calories, become more active, recognize emotional components of eating, and guide you into making changes in your eating environment.

"Weight management is a lifetime project..."

- Don't neglect the importance of the slow and steady approach. Weight management is a marathon, not a series of 100-yard dashes. Be wise and pace yourself through learning about your emotions, outside behavioral eating cues, and how to cope with various life situations that lead to improper eating. Make changes in your patterns slowly so they become second nature and you eventually won't have to think about eating healthy—it will be what you do naturally.
- Be patient! Weight management is a lifetime project—not one that is won or lost in three to six weeks. Perseverance usually wins out. Set realistic goals based on your body fat amount.
- Think positively and tell yourself that you will change habits little by little. Don't dwell on past failures. Favorite foods don't have to be entirely forbidden.
- Write down your goals, both short and long-term. Make sure they are realistic and attainable.

Mood Awareness

- Be aware of what you are putting in your mouth (and your mood at the time).
- Try not to eat when bored, tired, or depressed. Promise yourself that when you feel the urge to snack, you will do something else for at least thirty minutes (e.g. go for a walk, phone a friend, write a letter, etc.). If you eat out of boredom, find some new hobby or interest that gets you out of the house.
- Perform charting for awhile. This doesn't have to go on indefinitely, but for the next several weeks, weigh and measure food and drink intake. Look for *major eating trends,* in addition to the usual charting of fats and calories.
- Develop positive attitude *flash cards* and look at them several times a day. Condition your mind (and eventually your attitudes) by repeating key phrases over and over.
- Realize that eating is a behavior that is greatly influenced by people with whom we live or socialize, places where we find ourselves, and our own emotions. Know who your friends really are. Those who purposefully try to lure you from your desired weight program are not your true friends. In most cases, you would probably be better off without that kind of friendship.
- Think of eating as engine maintenance, not as a recreational sport.

"...eating is a behavior..."

Changes

- Once you have identified potentially problematic areas, pick a few key ones and begin to work on them. Eating breakfast, slower eating, smaller portions, bingeing, and social situations are all areas that most of us could use some improvement in.
- Ask others to help you, especially by not tempting you or snacking around you. By incorporating their help, you will feel more dedicated and they will be less likely to sabotage your efforts. Have them show their affection to you in non-food ways.
- Keep problematic foods out of sight, or better still, out of the house. Keep serving dishes off the table. Shop with a list when not hungry and read those labels.
- Plan ahead for social outings. Perhaps eat something partially filling before going out or at least limit high-fat foods and sauces and high calorie drinks.
- Build your self-esteem. How you feel about yourself affects so much of your life and what you can accomplish. Adopt a more positive and brighter outlook on life.
- As you progress on your weight management program, remember that you owe no one any explanation or apology for losing weight and improving your appearance and health.
- Look for habits you know deep inside need to be changed (e.g. eating quickly, large mouthfuls, eating when tense or bored, eating every bite on a plate even when not hungry, eating while distracted, etc.)

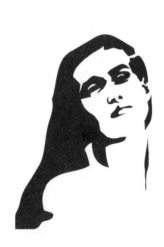

Long Term

- Don't even purchase problem high-calorie foods. Shop from a set list to prevent impulse buying and try to shop without children. Plan your meals well in advance and stick to a set menu.
- Plan ahead for social occasions in your mind and rehearse repeatedly what you will do in certain situations. Remind yourself several times daily that you are in charge of your actions and that you *can be* determined and strong willed.
- If food seems to dominate your life, look into professional counseling. At the very least, you may wish to consider joining a weight management group with regular meetings (e.g. Weight Watchers, Over Eaters Anonymous, TOPS). Work on this problem with a friend or spouse. Encourage each other.

"Plan ahead for social occasions..."

Other Considerations

DAILY MEALS

Consistent patterns are important in any weight management program. One of the best patterns that you can develop is to try to eat at least *three regular meals per day*. Studies of overweight people have shown that many obese people routinely skip breakfast, and many skip lunch too. Most of their eating is accomplished from supper until bedtime, yet they stay overweight. A partial explanation could be that they may have a higher tendency to binge (due to skipping meals) and to eat more at the meal(s) they do eat. They may not be practicing the principles of sound nutrition, which include *consistent* and *properly spaced* meals, as well as *specific* and *limited* eating places.

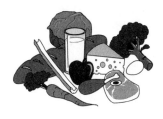

Eating at least three meals a day helps supply your body with a steady supply of fuel to maintain your basal metabolic rate. A higher basal (baseline) metabolic rate means more calories burned during the day. It may take several months to offset the metabolic reduction caused by chronic dieting—so be patient. By not skipping meals, you are also helping to neutralize improper *dieting thinking*. The calories saved by missing lunch could well show up by overeating at dinner due to an inflated appetite. Re-educate yourself and your eating habits by avoiding fad diets and by eating at least three nutritionally balanced meals daily.

"...the goal is to re-train ourselves towards proper eating..."

When you eat in a more normal, physiologic manner, along with gradual substitution of lowfat alternatives in these meals, you are positively shaping your lifestyle behavior away from dieting. When you eat a high-fiber breakfast, you may prevent a later mid-morning high-fat snack attack. Eat small frequent meals rather than one or two big meals. This is especially true if you have trouble with fatigue or low blood sugar symptoms (hypoglycemia). You will help rid yourself of the usual feelings of deprivation that can lead to loss of eating control.

A word to those who complain, "If I eat something for breakfast, I'm hungry all day long." As mentioned earlier, the goal is to re-train ourselves towards proper eating, not improper dieting. Our bodies are like machines and do need fuel all day long. If we supply the proper fuel in the form of multiple food fuelings, it should perform better. Try proper eating instead of improper dieting and see what it can do for you.

PLATEAU

The dictionary defines *plateau* as "an elevated and comparatively level expanse of land". Weight-reducers sometimes have more *colorful* descriptions of it. Whatever term you use, few things are more frustrating and mentally discouraging than attempting weight reduction, yet stepping on the scale day after day to find body weight *stuck* at one number.

This is where positive thinking and knowing what is happening physiologically becomes important. If we remember that we are undertaking *slow* and *deliberate* changes in our eating habits and lifestyle, and that our body needs time to adapt and make physiologic changes, then a plateau becomes something we *expect* from time to time — rather than dread.

During times of famine, the body makes automatic changes (such as metabolism reduction) in an attempt to conserve body integrity. Many other adaptive changes occur over time, including replacement of diminishing fat cell mass with increased tissue fluid. Such changes also occur and may last for *several weeks* during caloric restriction and attempts to reduce weight.

"Concentrate on health and a healthful appearance..."

Concentrate on health and a healthful appearance and not a specific weight on the scale. Realize that absolute weight may not tell the complete story of what is really happening. Those *increasing* their lean body weight through increased exercise may offset fat weight loss, thereby rendering the scale readings unimportant. Weight can remain stationary even though you are reproportioning body tissue mass and losing inches.

SUPPORT GROUPS

One factor which is highly correlated with maintenance of long-term weight loss is *social support*. This usually involves family and friends but can extend to workmates, business associates, and weight management groups. Support by other family members, particularly a spouse, was found to be one of the most important success factors for weight reducers.

Whatever the support, make a commitment to them and have them make a commitment to you. Once they do, they will be less likely to sabotage your efforts. This is especially true with a spouse or family member. Encourage each other and have them monitor your progress (this relates to your accountability). Having a reward system for you and them will keep the process interesting and help maintain it on a long-term basis. Set goals and rewards such as clothes, a favorite book or movie, a special holiday or something special to you.

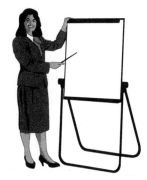

There are several weight management and support groups available in some communities. Weight Watchers, Overeaters Anonymous, Take Off Pounds Sensibly (TOPS), and hospital-based weight counseling are just a few of some groups that may be helpful. Each has its own merits, so you will need to be the judge which one(s) may benefit you.

TODAY'S LIFESTYLES

No book on weight management could be complete without due consideration to today's lifestyles and their impact on our health and weight. We might be puzzled why our weight creeps up on us until we stop to assess changes that have gradually occurred over the last several decades. One sign states that 'Overweight is something that just *snacks* up on you'. This addresses just one part of the weight equation. The other is seen in the decrease (usually subtle) in our daily activities.

The following article from *Prevention* captures the essence of the matter. It is up to us to find ways to reverse this trend. Besides suggestions in the article, see also the 'Exercise' and 'Activities of Daily Living' sections of this book.

Reprinted from PREVENTION

Let's Beat the Deficiency That Makes Us Fat!

Why is it so hard to stay slim? Most of the people I talk to swear they don't eat all that much. Most, in fact, are convinced they eat less than they did years ago—when they were 10, 20, even 40 or 50 pounds lighter than they are today.

It's my opinion that the biggest underlying cause of overweight is found in the title of the classic Charlie Chaplin film *Modern Times*.

What these modern times have done is create a huge deficiency—a deficiency of exercise, resulting in big-time "flabola."

Yes, despite the heralded interest in fitness walking, aerobics and all the rest, the average person today gets much less exercise than his counter-part did a generation or two ago. Back then, people got exercise just by living—living in the 1940s or '50s or even '60s instead of the 1990s.

"...the deficiency comes from lots of little things..."

Remarkably few people realize the extent of this deficiency, even when the result of it is staring at us from the snickering face of a bathroom scale. The tricky part is that the deficiency comes from lots of little things, so little they're nearly invisible. But look at this—a kind of split-screen image, with 1953 on the left side and 1993 on the right.

A Split-Screen View of Modern History

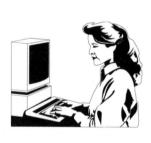

It's morning and Mrs. 1953 walks a few blocks (one-quarter mile) to the bus, as Mr. 1953 is using the one family car to drive to work. She has another quarter-mile walk to her office job on the second floor of a building with no elevator. Once ensconced at her desk, she seems to get precious little exercise, spending the day pounding away on an old Underwood.

Now, on the other side of the screen, let's look at Mrs. 1993. Hers is a two-car household, so she motors 15 minutes to work, then takes the elevator to the fifteenth floor, where she spends her day pounding the keyboard of a computer.

The difference doesn't seem so great, does it? After all, Mrs. 1953 wasn't working in a steel mill, and she climbed only one flight of stairs to reach her desk.

In fact, the difference is about 16 pounds. Yes, assuming they're the same size with the same metabolism and eat the same amount of food, just the part of Mrs. 1993's daily regimen we described will, in time, make her close to 16 pounds heavier.

That's because Mrs. 1953 burned 100 calories a day walking to and from her bus stops, and—believe it or not—about another 100 extra calories using a manual typewriter instead of an electronic keyboard. A few daily trips up and down the stairs at work (almost three minutes) burn about another 20 calories, for a total of 220 calories.

For roughly every 15 calories you stop burning on a daily basis while eating the same amount of food, you will in time get 1 pound heavier—for a total of 16 big ones in Mrs. 1993's case.

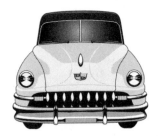

"...our contemporaries have a cellular..."

Meanwhile, her husband drives 30 minutes to work, just like his dad did 40 years ago. After a brief stop at the office, he goes out on the street, where he's a salesman driving through city traffic for about three hours a day, just like his dad did.

Difference? Nearly *12 pounds*.

But how could that be? Simple. Mr. 1993 has an automatic shift, while his dad, driving a stick, actually burned an additional 140 calories a day.

Interesting, huh?

But that's just the beginning.

Because they're a two-job family, our modern couple eats out three nights a week. Over on the left side of the screen, our '50s couple ate out just once a week.

Difference? For whoever does the kitchen work, about *another 5 pounds*. That's the result of not preparing dinner twice a week. Plus, I forgot to mention that our modern couple has a dishwasher!

Come late evening, our '50s couple liked to watch their new TV, though Mr. 1953 used to pop up 15 times a night to fiddle with the aerial or change the channel. Our modern-times guy just sits there with his thumb resting on the remote.

And while Mrs. 1953 usually did knitting while she watched the mostly boring shows on Stone Age TV, our modern woman is completely enthralled with the vivid images on her 27-inch Sony. Besides, she doesn't know how to knit.

Difference, *probably about 2 pounds each*. Plus, *1 more pound* can probably be tacked on because, instead of scampering to get the phone (in the kitchen) every time it rings, our contemporaries have a cellular that's always in reach.

Come weekends, Mr. 1953 did yard work. So does his son in 1993. But while Dad spent an hour and a half at a shot pushing a mower over the homestead, sonny boy uses a riding mower and is done in 20 minutes. Difference? At 20 mows a year, *over 4 pounds*.

When the snows came in Elmira, New York—where Mr. 1953 lived—he'd shovel his steps, pathway and sidewalk all by hand, about a 600-calorie job. Junior, like so many moderns, lives in the Sunbelt. At 10 no-snows per year, he's just gained *2 more pounds*.

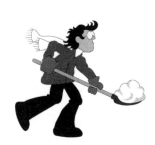

"...we all drive to shopping centers and malls."

Both like to use hand tools, though, for pruning trees, preparing firewood and making little projects. But—you guessed it— while dear old Dad burned 390 calories brandishing a handsaw for an hour, Junior uses a power saw and does the same amount of work in five minutes. Result after a year of sawing and puttering (about 25 hours' worth): *3 more pounds* on the young 'un's belly.

Back in the '50s, our couple frequently took short walks to the grocery store, fish store, butcher shop, library, drugstore and dry cleaner. Today, the vast majority of these little shops no longer exist, and we all drive to shopping centers and malls. Carry a bag of groceries two or three blocks? Who does that anymore (except in New York City)? You can probably slap on *another 6 pounds*. By now, it's likely that our modern couple is a good 50 pounds heavier (combined weight) than their '50s counterparts. Even if they eat considerably less food, they'll still be noticeably plumper. But we're not through yet.

Consider the modern automobile, not with just auto shift (which we accounted for previously), but also with power steering, power brakes, cruise control, power windows, power door locks, even a power aerial. Back in 1953, most cars didn't even

"You just sit for hours in front of a computer..."

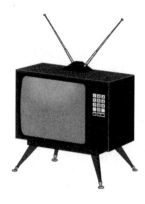

"...we're way past sedentary..."

have turn signals—you had to roll down the window and make arcane hand signals. All that (especially the power steering) is probably worth *another 2 pounds*.

Take the modern workstation, where it's unnecessary to get up and search out bulky files from cabinets and shelves. You just sit for hours in front of a computer, seeking and processing with mere taps of the fingers. You can probably chuck on *2 more pounds*.

The very design of modern homes makes us fatter. Many of us who were raised in vertical homes now live in ranches. No more up and down the stairs 10 times a day.

No more running up and down and about to open and shut windows—the automatic climate control takes care of all our temperature needs.

And appliances.

Who kneads dough by hand anymore? Or stirs a thick batter by spoon, when there are automated ways of doing just about everything except peeling a banana?

And the lure of the TV, the VCR and the PC, not to mention the CD-ROM.

There's even don't-get-up-and-change-the-record-you-might-burn-a-calorie multidisc CD players.

How to Cure Virtual Immobility

We used to hear that modern lifestyles were becoming sedentary. Well, we're way past sedentary now and into virtual *immobility*.

You could turn on a motion-detector alarm system in a modern household with four people in it, and the thing wouldn't go off until someone had to visit the bathroom.

So there it is.

Because we are now in the dawn of what I call the Age of Akinesis (total lack of human movement), we are paying the price in pounds. And I don't mean British sterling.

All the normal, everyday, no-big-deal ways we used to burn calories and keep slim are gone forever. Think about that: forever.

There is, of course, no turning back the clock. If anything, the speed of change is increasing.

That's why we believe that creating an exercise program for yourself is the best and perhaps only way to prevail over an environment automated to the point of biological toxicity. You know, fat really is toxic, greasing the skids for most of the major health threats we face today. What's more, *not* exercising is itself toxic, now recognized as a major risk factor for heart disease.

Put those two facts together, and the motive for regenerating your physical vitality is mighty strong.

NOTE: All calculations are based on a 150-pound person. Numbers will vary from person to person based on amount of regular exercise, diet and other factors.

Food Diary

One of the most important lifestyle behaviors that can be stressed is *self-monitoring*. Part of such supervision involves a journal or diary. If you are tempted to lightly skip over this recommendation, look upon this as a cornerstone of behavior modification.

First of all, to change or modify inappropriate or unhealthy behavior, one must first become *aware of* and *identify* such behavior. The food, mood, exercise, and fluid-intake diary becomes this identification tool.

"Recording in detail will heighten your awareness..."

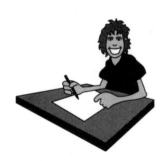

Secondly, nationwide surveys of persons experiencing the greatest success with weight reduction typically were those who utilized diaries. Self-monitoring, of which diaries can play an important part, has been shown to be a primary factor in successful long-term weight maintenance after reducing.

How long you continue such monitoring is up to you. In general, the longer the better. Use it to identify and correct non-productive behavior and eating patterns. While calories and amount of activity are important guidelines, you should concentrate on finding *patterns* in these areas.

Recording in detail will heighten your awareness of eating, associated moods or triggers to eating, and your true amount of activity (or lack thereof). It forces your attention to focus on areas that may need change. Once awareness is gained, it can become a key to changing unwanted habits or reinforcing appropriate ones.

One study tracked nine women and one man who reported failing to lose weight after many attempts at dieting. The study showed that these self-proclaimed *diet-resistant* people actually *underreported* the amount of food eaten by an average of 47 percent and *overreported* their physical activity by 51 percent. Analysis of the data showed that the errors made by the participants may have been unintentional. There was probably a certain amount of denial involved. It is probable that if they had eaten as little and been as active as they thought, they would have lost weight.

Even a group of subjects who were not overweight underreported their calorie intake by about 20%. Perhaps poor weight loss in the past that has been attributed to *slow metabolism* may really be due to *calorie amnesia*.

A multitude of benefits can be derived by record keeping for those attempting weight modification. Some of these include the following:

- **Helps with food choices:**
  —Encourages meal planning. Try making meal plans for a week at a time. Avoid spontaneous or random eating experiences.
  —Identifies hidden fats and excessive calories.
  —Problem foods and beverages can be highlighted.

- **Puts you in a position of control:**
  —Gives a running assessment of daily allotment.
  —Allows your discretion to allow additional intake.
  —Helps bolster self-control, especially when diary checked by support person on a regular basis.

- **Simplifies and identifies eating patterns:**
  —Shows meals skipped.
  —Pinpoints eating throughout the day or while doing something else.
  —Major consumption from supper until bedtime (very common in obese individuals).
  —Moods, feelings, and situations—identify relationship to eating.

- **Prevents *calorie amnesia*:**
  —"What was the exact number of chips consumed at the party?"
  —"How many ounces of juice did you drink at breakfast?"

- **Encourages activity and exercise:**
  —Documents increase in *activities of daily living*—positive feedback.
  —Points out deficiencies and opportunities for being more active.

- **Progress assessment tool for your doctor, dietitian or counselor.**

"Record everything and forget nothing."

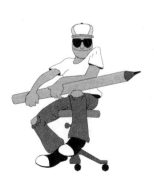

Use a food diary similar to **Example 1** which follows. Many such diaries are available in booklet form. You do not have to get fancy—a memo book used to write down the day, time, item eaten and quantity, general mood, and activity will suffice. Always carry the food record and record *immediately* after eating. Do not wait until the next day or night before you see your physician or counselor to make your records. These records can be transferred to a larger notebook or diary at the end of the day—at which time you can total fats, calorie intake, and/or calorie expenditure. Look for fat intake, calories, activity, moods, and trends. Let the diary serve *you*. Don't be enslaved by it!

At least for a few days, try to include every *time* and every *thing* you eat—from colas to cheese, milk to mangos, or beer to bubblegum. Record everything and forget nothing. Every ounce of food and beverage should be entered, especially until you become familiar with portion sizes. If you decide why you are eating, you start to isolate some of the urges behind your own eating behavior. Be aware of those times and situations when *true* hunger is not the primary driving force for eating.

If you are focusing on calorie restriction, watch your fat intake as well. Any *calorie counting* program should be a *fat counting* program as well. Utilize your diary to monitor whether you are eating enough bulky *basic nutrient* foods requiring some sort of preparation and *less* empty, refined, processed and ready-to-eat higher calorie food items.

EXAMPLE 1

"You do not have to get fancy...a memo book...will suffice."

"Look for fat intake, calories, activity, moods, and trends."

SAMPLE FOOD DIARY

Day: Thursday (2/14)

Time/Place/Mood	ITEM Eaten	Quantity	Calories	Fats
Breakfast —McDonalds —felt tired	Apple Bran Muffin	1	190	0 gm
10:00 am —office —depressed	Donut	1	235	13gm
Lunch —home —calm	Green beans Hamburger helper	1/2 c. 1 serv.	22 350	0 gm 16gm

(Total Calories and Fats for the day):

Activities today: *watched tv, vacuumed and swept, office work*

Exercise: *fifteen minute walk at lunch—moderate pace*

General Mood:

Eating Control: Poor 1 2 ③ 4 5 Good

Assertiveness

The following questions and journal will help you to assess your assertiveness. Since many of us find ourselves pressured to give in to the party host, the well-meaning spouse, or *mom* at that special holiday, this exercise may enlighten you as to some of your strengths and weaknesses. As part of our ultimate goal of awareness of eating, behavior, moods, and attitudes, it should help to illuminate this aspect of your personality.

Answer each question with only one of the three numbers to indicate which one of them best describes your *present* behavior. Each number is used as follows:

—ONE (1) means 'NO' or *almost never.*
—TWO (2) means *some of the time only* or *average.*
—THREE (3) means *usually always* or *practically every time.*

"...many of us find ourselves pressured to give in..."

Please be honest with your responses. You are the only one that will see the results. Add up the totals in each column. Next, add up the totals of all three columns. A low score of **33** indicates an almost total lack of assertiveness in situations involving your weight control effort. A maximum possible score of **99** indicates an excellent degree of assertiveness in standing up for your rights to be thin. Scores in between these two extremes will give you a fairly good idea of where you stand in regards to the need for improvement.

On each line, write-in either number 1, 2, or 3. Write the number in the proper column to match the number at the top of that column.

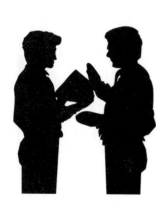

	1	2	3
1. If you are standing in a cafeteria line, do you protest and speak up when someone gets in front of you?			
2. At a buffet or cocktail party, are you the first to introduce yourself and begin a conversation with a stranger?			
3. When someone makes an unfair criticism about your weight control effort, do you call it to his/her attention?			
4. Do you find it generally easy to express what you feel at the moment?			
5. Do you feel undisturbed and at ease when other people watch you eat?			
6. If someone keeps kicking you or bumping you under the dinner table, do you ask that person to stop?			
7. When you have a meal with friends, do you find it easy to control the conversation?			
8. Is it easy for you to refuse second helpings, desserts, or other foods you don't want?			
9. When discussing diets with another person, are you able to speak up for your own viewpoint?			
10. When someone presses you to have a drink with them, do you find it easy to refuse?			
11. Do you feel comfortable when not wanting to explain why you wish to eat only certain food at a party?			
12. Is it easy for you to make decisions about proper choices in front of other people?			

	1	2	3

13. Do you ordinarily have confidence in your own judgment when deciding on a specific eating behavior? ....

14. If someone criticizes you about your obesity, are you able to respond in a calm and collected manner? ....

15. Are you able to refuse unreasonable requests from friends, if such would interfere with your reducing effort? ....

16. Can you praise or compliment another person easily when you feel they deserve it? ....

17. Are you reluctant to speak up in a debate or discussion about dieting and weight reduction? ....

18. When a meal in a prestigious restaurant is not prepared as you ordered, do you ask the waiter to correct it? ....

19. Can you deal effectively with persons who repeatedly attempt to embarrass you about your weight problem? ....

20. When you find a suit or dress you bought is too small for you, do you return it for an adjustment? ....

21. Are you able to express affection and love openly to someone who has helped you with weight control? ....

22. Do you insist that other family members take on a fair share of the cooking responsibilities? ....

23. When a latecomer's table is served before yours in a restaurant, do you call attention to the situation? ....

24. If it is vital to your weight control effort, are you able to ask friends for help or favors? ....

25. If someone has borrowed one of your diet books and is overdue in returning it, do you mention it? ....

26. Are you openly critical when someone in a group is obviously giving erroneous nutritional information? ....

27. Can you calmly defend your position when someone tries to tell you "you are losing weight the wrong way?" ....

28. Do you reply without name-calling or obscenities when you are angered by negative remarks about your figure? ....

29. When someone belittles your repeated dieting attempts, do you respond in a rational manner? ....

30. Do you find it easy to refuse a special dish recommended by a waiter if you'd rather choose something else? ....

31. If someone eats one of your favorite but forbidden foods in front of you, do you tell him/her it disturbs you? ....

32. Without shouting, can you tell members of your household to avoid bringing certain foods into the house? ....

33. When asked to attend a social function laden with tempting foods, can you say *no* without feeling guilty? ....

Enter total score for each of the columns at bottom of that column ....

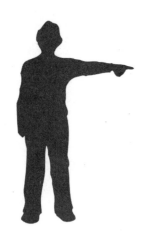

"...are you able to ask friends for help..."

Copyright © 1977 by American Society of Bariatric Physicians.
Assertiveness material by Peter G. Lindner, M.D.
Reproduced by permission.

TIP: If you would like help with assertiveness, try a book entitled "*When I Say No, Why Do I Feel Guilty?*" by Manuel Smith.

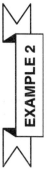

EXAMPLE 2

Copyright © 1977 by American Society of Bariatric Physicians. Reproduced by permission.

This is a sample assertiveness chart you can make for yourself to help you in future food encounters.

Assertivenss Journal

WEIGHT CONTROL RELATED SITUATION	SYMPTOMS	BEHAVIOR	EMOTION	DESIRES	REASON	FUTURE ASSERTIVE TECHNIQUE
Describe in detail what actually occurred; include what other person actually said; also give date.	Physical effects I noticed.	How I responded; what I did.	How I felt at the time of incident.	What I wanted to do.		Describe technique you plan to use in the future; write down words you will use.
Example of Typical Entry Hostess offered me my favorite cake and said that she made it just for me. I was at a party with 10 other people. Date: July 4th, 1987.	Heart beating rapidly; voice tense; mouth watering in expectation.	After one refusal I agreed to *just one small piece*. Turned out to be 2 pieces. It was just too good.	Frustrated, felt trapped. Felt I was a failure on my weight control effort.	Tell her that I did not want to eat any, without having to explain why.	Afraid of offending hostess and hurting her feelings. Also, have other people make fun of my dietary attempts.	*Parrot Technique:* "No, thank you, I don't want any!" Repeat saying this over and over without giving any reason for my decision. It's my right not to have to explain reasons for my behavior.
			—FILL IN YOUR OWN SPECIFICS HERE—			

Behavior Modification

Behavior modification is a cornerstone in the foundation of successful weight reduction and management. It is based on the idea that daily habits should be changed in order to promote long-term weight control. By use of food diaries or other techniques, adverse behaviors are recognized and replaced with healthier attitudes, actions, or eating and activity patterns.

Part of the modification recommended by this program involves substitutions—lower fat foods for those with high-fat and increased activity for inactivity. Seek ways to reduce food and food cue exposure. Special occasions, certain times of the day, or even certain smells may evoke unwanted behavior and must be handled in a positive way.

"Part of the modification ...involves substitutions..."

Components of successful behavior change include:
- *identification* of lifestyle or eating pattern needing change
- *modification* of causes of the undesired behavior utilizing problem solving, contingency planning, and visualization
- behavioral *goals* that are specific, realistic, and gradually implemented
- positive *reinforcement* of desired behavior utilizing non-food rewards

In order to produce permanent eating pattern changes that become second nature, a *gradual* change of habits to a healthier, lower fat eating style is recommended. Start with one meal or one food at a time. Reduce the item(s) with the most fat or most saturated fat first. Half of your usual portion size would be an excellent place to begin. As you begin limiting certain items, *phase in* recipe substitutions to counter any feelings of deprivation.

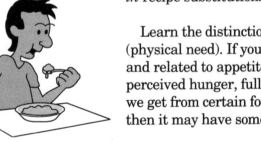

Learn the distinction between *appetite* (psychological need) and true hunger (physical need). If your *mouth* needs something, it's probably just a food craving and related to appetite. Appetite consists of conscious sensations including perceived hunger, fullness, food cravings, and the pleasure and 'good feelings' we get from certain foods. However, if your *stomach* is aching or seems hollow, then it may have some hunger component.

It is often cited that appetite will resolve within twenty minutes or so, whether you empty the cookie jar or not. This is used to justify recommending alternatives to eating as a substitute when you think you are hungry, especially between meals. Many overweight people rank eating fifth or lower on a scale of priorities (though individual variations do occur). If you make your own *substitution* list—such as those listed below—with activities that are *equally* or *more enjoyable* to you than eating, you will be well on your way to conquering your weight problem.

Keep the list in descending order. That is, put your most enjoyable activity at the top of the list and so on. Make sure you list things which you could actually do on a regular basis. A trip to Europe might be nice, but certainly couldn't be used as a substitute each time you had inappropriate food cravings.

Do things on your list which you have placed higher than eating whenever you feel yourself wanting to snack or overeat.

GOOD FOOD SUBSTITUTES:

Call or stop in to see a friend or neighbor.

Write a long-overdue letter to the editor, a governmental official, or a friend.

Go to the public library, read a good book, or flip through a magazine.

Rent a video, go see a movie, or listen to an old record, tape, or CD.

Plan your next vacation, mini-weekend getaway, or time off.

Do a word-search or crossword puzzle.

Paint a T-shirt or picture.

Cross-stitch, crochet, sew, or other hand work.

Work on a hobby or small project.

Work in the garden, pick flowers, prune shrubs or bushes.

Take a walk, hike, bike ride, or other physical activity.

Organize photos in an album or just take a trip down memory lane.

Join a club or volunteer organization.

Tend to the pets (walk dog, clean fish tank, etc.).

Pick flowers, rake leaves, edge lawn.

Clean out a drawer or two.

Rearrange a room or start planning for redecorating it.

Take a nap or go to bed early.

Play a game with the kids or talk with them about their day.

Read a daily devotional.

Take a drive somewhere.

Go window shopping.

Balance your checkbook.

Clean out and organize your purse or wallet.

Organize and polish your shoes.

Re-read this book.

Awareness & Attitudes

Before delving further into the importance of attitude in weight management, it must be mentioned that self-worth and appearance are not necessarily interconnected. Both may influence each other, but each and every individual is special in their own right.

"...become conscious of what is going on."

Long-term successful weight management seems to work best as a *partnership*. As part of this patient-counselor partnership, each must accept shared responsibility toward a lifelong commitment to needed changes in lifestyle, behavior, and dietary practices.

Of prime importance is how to identify *needed changes*, such as unperceived urges to eat. One step is to *become conscious* of what is going on. Attention to our eating must become focused, similar to eyeglasses focusing blurry images to make things clear. We will then be able to see with greater clarity our feelings, our minds, and our bodies. This puts us in contact with who we really are and what is really going on.

We have to depart from being *double-minded* in respect to dieting. In the old view, dieters and foods were either good or bad. Since people are not perfect, when someone did eventually *slip*, they placed themselves in the

"...there are no forbidden foods!"

terrible (or bad) category. This led to feelings of inadequacy and low self-esteem, which further compounded the problem.

Realize, there are no forbidden foods! None that are legal or illegal. By the way, how did you feel when you just read these sentences? Unbelieving? Skeptical? Like a two-ton burden had just been lifted from your shoulders?

What happens when the *pressure to perform* is removed? Usually a wonderful new feeling of freedom. You are in control. You are now allowed to view eating as a matter of *choices*, not deprivations!

Of course, realistic choices for most people with weight problems will not include eating anything and everything *all the time*. Intelligent and smart thinkers will start looking for alternatives to *gradually substitute* for improper foods and behaviors, thereby replacing unhealthy ones.

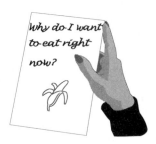

How does one bring something to conscious awareness? The food diary is mentioned elsewhere in this book and may be reviewed at this time. Another way is through the use of placards, self-notes, or posters placed strategically throughout the house (pantry, refrigerator, cupboard, cookie jars or other countertop food containers) or office. On these posters, you can place pictures of healthy foods and activities or questions like, "Am I truly hungry right this minute?" or "*Why* do I want to eat right now?"

The purpose of such notes is to make our conscious mind *aware* of these eating cues and habits. From there it will be transferred to our subconscious. Once aware of overeating, weight gain, or deviation from our desired behavior modification, we can activate our problem solving routines. Eventually we will then re-program our subconscious with healthier attitudes and choices, but this requires repetition, hence the numerous notes and posters.

The actual behavior of eating has many cues and controls. Our emotions are but one of these. Our friends, relatives, acquaintances, and co-workers also have input. Situations (places, sites, social events) impact our behavior too, so be aware of ones that lead to extra food intake. So many people eat to temporarily reduce tension and release pressure.

"We must plan in advance..."

We must plan in advance how to counter nibbling *danger times*, especially those emotionally triggered or due to stress, depression, boredom, or fatigue. Know *before* the temptation occurs what you will do. Simple suggestions include hand-mind occupying activity, taking walks, or relaxation exercises.

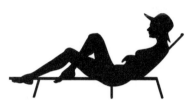

RELAXATION: There are several types of relaxation exercises. The following are just a few. One suggested technique is to find a quiet area, lean back in a recliner or on a bed. Close your eyes and starting at your head or foot, purposely tense muscles in that area for several seconds, then relax them. Then move down (or up) until you have covered your entire body. Don't forget eyes, face, stomach, thighs, calves, and chest. A variation of this technique is to picture hot oil being poured on your head. As the thick, hot oil gently runs down over each part of your body, picture it warming and relaxing the muscles in that area.

Another relaxation technique is to relax in a comfortable place (as above), close your eyes, and concentrate on your breathing. Take in a deep breath, picture it completely filling your lungs, and hold it for three or four seconds. Then let it out very slowly. Take a couple of regular breaths and then repeat with the deep breath that you hold for several seconds. Repeat this cycle for eight to ten times as you picture tension and stress leaving your body each time you slowly exhale. Some people like to picture a color that represents tension and stress to them. They visualize their body being filled with this color at the start. Each time they slowly exhale, they picture the color being expelled along with the breath. As the color fades, so will the tension.

How does one cope with feelings of guilt about eating high-calorie food, which may lead to further eating or bingeing? A start would be to focus on positives rather than negatives. Tell yourself that favorite foods are not absolutely forbidden and that your plan is to change habits in small increments (little by little). Many healthy weight maintainers have been successful by not forbidding themselves controlled amounts of some of their favorite foods.

"Eat smaller servings of foods you wish to limit."

Weight will be lost if you focus on small changes consistently versus large changes inconsistently. As for eating high-fat, high-calorie foods — gradually substitute lower-fat, lower-calorie foods. Eat smaller servings of foods you wish to limit. Reduce alcohol, caffeine and refined sugar intake. Eat more fruits, vegetables, and whole grain items. You *do not* have to make all these changes at once. Like any good project, break it down into smaller parts.

One roadblock that some may face is truly believing that attitudes towards food and coping strategies can be changed long-term. You can acquire help in this area by utilizing individualized, positive self-statements that are written down and periodically read (perhaps eight to ten times a day). Make up your own but for starters try: "I am in control," "It's okay to be myself," "I choose to be free of hunger (appetite)," "I can stay on my eating plan and lose weight," "I can be more active today than yesterday," or "It's okay to leave food on my plate." Stay with one until you tire of it, then switch to a new one.

Such *positive affirmation* will burn these powerful thoughts into your subconscious mind. They will then become available when you need them most. Try it, even if you are skeptical right now.

Situations

Even when we are not really hungry, some situations and circumstances tend to make us eat. Besides hunger, situational stimuli and emotional upset are powerful motivators for eating. Situations lead us into stimuli that evoke extra food intake.

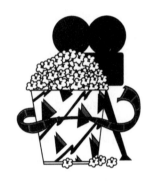

"...food contacts... up to twenty a day!"

How many of us are tempted by the popcorn and candy at the movies, the chips and dip at the party, or the cocktail peanuts on the bar? Just the *sight* of some foods in certain situations can trigger eating. This is one place a food diary can make us more aware of these triggers and can help to slow down inappropriate pre-programmed responses.

Do we eat food for the same reasons some mountaineers climb mountains — because it's there? Is the food tempting to look at or smell? Do we eat just to be sociable when everyone else seems to be doing it? Surveys say an *average* person daily eats three meals and six or seven snacks. Children before age 12 and women ages 25 to 44 were found to be snackers with the most food contacts — up to 20 a day!

Obviously, true hunger is not the motivation behind all this nibbling. Besides the aforementioned situational stimuli, even emotional upsets can become cues to satisfy ourselves with food. Doldrums, despair, restlessness, guilt, apprehension, frustration, stress, anger, or isolation may cause us to tackle the strawberry-shortcake instead of tackling the problem.

Use of food to relieve situational urges and emotional distress is often unconscious. If we respond to these stimuli every time they arise, food intake becomes excessive.

How does one cope with eating high-calorie food just because its offered or because others around are eating it? Start by realizing your limitations and ask for help. You may request that no one offer you food, others not snack or nibble around you, and people show fondness for you in non-food related ways.

If visual cues tempt you into eating high-calorie foods, keep the food out of sight. Everyone remembers the phrase, "Out of sight, out of mind." It

"Out of sight, out of mind, and out of mouth!"

could be revised to include, "Out of sight, out of mind, and out of mouth!" By shopping with a list and on a full stomach, you can start by not buying high-calorie foods and beverages. Even if you do, *hide them* in inconvenient, out-of-the-way places out of sight. Do not serve meals family style by leaving serving dishes on the table. Remove them from view immediately. Clean plates directly into the garbage or place in opaque containers.

Are social occasions a tough situational stimuli for you? Holiday parties, banquets, church suppers, and family reunions can totally sabotage your program unless you can bring your own supply of food. Plan ahead of time what you will eat –or– eat before you actually attend (soup, fruits, vegetable snack, etc.). Plan to consume (or even bring with you) lowfat, low-calorie foods and beverages or mixers. Ordering a-la-carte allows you to make alternative selections and limit intake. You might even wish to attend the function after the food is served or leave before if food is the last program item.

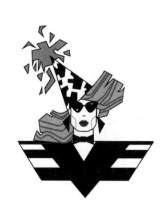

Do your best not to go to a social event hungry. A fruit and lots of fluid ahead of time will take the edge off your hunger. If someone offers you something not on your program, try telling them, "I'm full now, perhaps a little later." If you just tell them "no", you might be in for an explanation or argument, whereas "later" leaves little to argue with.

Social events are good examples of where visual imagery and strategy planning ahead of time comes in handy. As you picture the scenario of a social event, birthday party, or business trip, you can rehearse coping tactics. Several times before the event, imagine yourself eating the *new way* you have selected: e.g., ordering clear soup or salad, grilled chicken or fish, skipping dessert and just ordering coffee. The more you picture this event ahead of time, the easier it will be to follow-through when it occurs in real life.

"...you can rehearse coping tactics."

Just as we encourage our children to role-play and plan strategies ahead of time (withstanding peer pressure, drugs, sex), so must we repeatedly rehearse in our mind what we will do when confronted with improper eating situations and cues. Frequently remind yourself that you are in charge and can be strong-willed. Look for additional strategy training or guidance from friends or professionals.

Sites & Stimuli

In the same vein as situational stimuli, certain places (sites) evoke eating behavior. Many of us have eating habits related to *location*. Frank never takes a second drink unless he is at a party. Mary never eats dessert unless dining out. Sally will not eat popcorn unless at the movies (and

"Avoid visually-attractive foods."

then she needs it with butter topping). Bread and butter? Not for Harry except at business luncheons. Pastries? Janice never touches them except when she is at her mother's house.

Is this mere coincidence? Perhaps not. Studies have shown actual physiological changes in the body, such as insulin shifts, due to various environmental cues. We can help to minimize these cues by visualization techniques mentioned previously.

In order to reduce exposure to high-fat, high-calorie foods around the house (often a very problematic site), one should avoid tasting foods while cooking, shopping when not hungry, and shop only from a list. You should also try to buy only food requiring preparation.

The designated eating site is one of the best behavioral techniques to develop. Assigning a specific and limited eating area, as well as consistency and proper meal spacing becomes our goal. The eating area should be one constant location you have stipulated for *all of your eating*. You may even wish to mark it with a placemat on which you have written something like, "I only eat here. When I am here I only eat." When stimuli arise, ask yourself, "Am I really hungry enough to stop what I'm doing, get the food and take it to my eating place?" Many times the answer will be no.

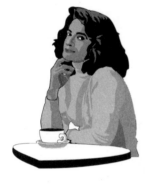

After several times of making the conscious decision not to interrupt yourself, you will begin to make it more subconsciously. This begins to free you from the urges of eating that you did not really want or need.

Even when triggered by certain sites or stimuli, we must localize and isolate true hunger. Do you really feel hunger in the pit of your stomach, or is it your mouth (taste buds) craving *something special*? If you are truly hungry, go to your designated *eating place* immediately. Take with you only as much food as you really want to eat and sit down. Utilizing proper eating utensils and dishes, eat there and nowhere else.

"When eating, do nothing else."

Avoid visually-attractive foods. Food companies pay thousands of dollars to market their products. One of their biggest expenditures is in the preparation and packaging of their product. When they go to so much trouble to make a food *seem irresistible*, you can almost bet that it *should* be avoided. The worse culprits are those that entice you to eat regardless of whether you are hungry or not. Be aware of these and keep them *out* of your home because they contain built-in cues to eat.

When eating, do nothing else. Eat in one room and in one chair. Avoid listening to the radio, watching TV or reading at the same time. The problem with eating while doing other activities is that these other activities start to become *associated with* hunger and eating in our minds. In these examples, the radio, TV, or book becomes a trigger to eat since we have *paired* it many times with the pleasurable experience of eating. Add to this other things we pair food with, such as sporting events, talking on the telephone, or playing cards, and you begin to get an idea of the multitude of *hunger cues* we impose upon ourselves.

If you are distracted by activities (such as were just mentioned), nibble while cooking, munch while walking around the house with food, or snack absentmindedly while holding the refrigerator door open, you may miss out on the *oral gratification* that your food should supply. This may lead to eating more than you wish. Eating at the eating spot forces attention towards the *ritual* of eating.

"...avoid the kitchen whenever possible."

The *kitchen* is one site that causes almost universal eating stimuli. A primary rule is to avoid the kitchen whenever possible. Only venture in when you *must* prepare meals or clean up afterwards. While there, keep foods (especially tempting ones) out of sight. Remove serving dishes quickly, scrape plates and deal with leftovers expeditiously, and keep food in opaque containers. It's best not to have problematic foods and beverages in the house, much less in the kitchen.

Reducing tempting stimuli should involve participation by family members. Ask that the not snack in front of you or offer you food. Have them express their love for you in other ways.

The office can be another site of frequent unwanted eating stimuli. The traditional *office coffee break* may encourage snacking, particularly on high-fat items such as pastries and donuts. One answer may be to *skip* the coffee break altogether by bringing your own thermos of coffee and having an alternative *enjoyment break*. This enjoyment could be routine or something different each day—walking, reading, writing, puzzles, handwork, vacation planning, etc. Another answer could be to bring fruits or lowfat, low-calorie alternatives to the donuts and pastries.

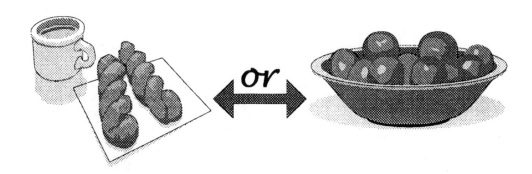

Habits & Emotions

Compulsive Overeating

When food is used in an *addictive* manner to symptomatically cope with feelings of anxiety, depression, or melancholy, this can point to being a symptom of compulsive overeating behavior. Inability to refrain from eating, even when not physically hungry, can also be a warning flag. Additional symptoms can include *preoccupation* with food, eating, weight, and diets.

Though there is some controversy as to the reasons people compulsively eat, several theories have been developed. People who compulsively eat may be trying to utilize food to try to *fill* an emptiness inside. It may be used as a self-soothing activity that provides substitute gratification for lost or disappointing love objects.

Food may also be used as a *diversion* against awareness of other uncomfortable or unacceptable feelings. One needs to realize that compulsive overeating and impulsive eating are addictions, just like other types of addictions.

"Food is used for its calming and sedating effects."

In this form of overeating disorder, eating is done impulsively, being triggered by *emotional* signals rather than *physical hunger*. Many times, the person involved cannot (or does not) distinguish true body feedback signals due to blocking out everything, including emotions. Food is used for its *calming* and *sedating* effects.

As children grow up, they usually respond to internal signals that tell them when they are full and when to stop eating. Some families may not encourage recognition and development of these *satiety signals*. Parents may encourage them to ignore these signals by focusing on emotional rather than physiologic cues. They may use food as a reward, for being good or calming down, or to help them with anxiety or tension.

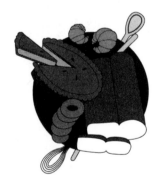

Persons with these behaviors that are attempting to lose weight just through dieting are setting themselves up for long-term failure. This is because the basic emotional issues and distorted body image problems are not addressed and corrected by traditional diets or diet programs. Treatment has to focus on changing many aspects of their lifestyle, not merely concentrating on losing weight or just the emotional aspects of the eating disorder.

The compulsive overeater can gain some benefit from using satiety strategies, oral gratification techniques, and slowing down the rate of eating. Many overeaters cannot handle *feeling empty* because when they do, that's when something triggers and the binges occur. Compulsive overeaters cannot stop at one potato chip or one cookie. The whole bag is at risk.

By only eating once or twice daily, they set themselves up to trigger the feast-famine cycle. Instead, they should use other low-calorie alternatives *throughout* the day as snacks and/or additional meals.

Oral gratification techniques are based on the premise that many urges to eat are not triggered by true hunger. Instead, the urge can be suppressed by alternatives

"Overeaters tend to gulp down food rapidly..."

(e.g. chewing on a toothpick or sugarless gum, sucking on a cinnamon stick, etc.). If the urge can be put off for 20 to 30 minutes, it will usually pass.

Overeaters tend to gulp down food rapidly, many times not even taking the extra time to really savor and enjoy it. Since the stomach may not send a *full signal* to the brain for at least 20 minutes after eating, eating too fast causes excessive food to be consumed before the full button is reached. If you feel you are a compulsive overeater, get professional help. You may also want to use many of the suggestions and slowing techniques mentioned elsewhere in this book.

Research continues into food cravings. Results so far indicate that eating fats or sweets causes the body to produce opioids (pleasure chemicals in the brain). Even chocolate has been found to contain a chemical that is just one side-chain different than the very addictive drug amphetamine.

Bad Habits

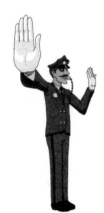

As mentioned earlier, in weight management one should get away from the concept of *good* vs. *bad* foods and habits. There are no such things as good foods and bad foods—just adequate and inadequate diets. It's how you select various foods that compose the total diet that really matters. We must think in terms of having a goal, and that goal may be to lose excess weight and be healthier. Things we do (and eat) will either be *productive* or *nonproductive* towards meeting that goal. It is the nonproductive things that many people consider *bad*, e.g. eating quickly, large mouthfuls, emotional eating, cleaning a plate because of childhood training, and the like.

We will list some nonproductive problems along with some productive plans to assist you. These will not be exhaustive lists but should supplement suggestions found elsewhere in this book.

PROBLEM: Eating while involved in other activities (reading, watching TV).
PLAN: Eat only and not during the activity. Consume food at your designated eating spot, not at the refrigerator or while standing.

PROBLEM: Eating high-fat, high-calorie foods.
PLAN: Select lower-fat, lower-calorie foods and substitute these gradually. Eat more carbohydrates (fruits, vegetables, whole grains) and less simple sugars. Reduce portion sizes of foods you desire to limit and consume less alcohol.

PROBLEM: Eating out of boredom, depression, or fatigue.
PLAN: Find a new hobby or interest, especially one that gets you out of the house (including adult education classes), do relaxation exercises, take walks, etc.

"Find a new hobby or interest..."

PROBLEM: Eating more than expected on social occasions.
PLAN: Decide upon a strategy ahead of time and determine what lower calorie items you will eat and drink. Rehearse repeatedly exactly what you will do and eat. Remind yourself of your strong will and determination to succeed. Eat before going out. Order a-la-carte.

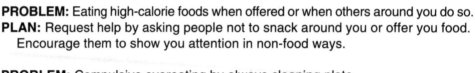

PROBLEM: Impulse to snack.
PLAN: Participate in some activity that will distract you from food. Take a walk, write a letter, or telephone a friend.

PROBLEM: Eating when you see tempting high-calorie food.
PLAN: Keep food out of view. Hide tempting foods—place in opaque, hard-to-reach containers. Do not keep serving dishes on the table or easily accessible during meals.

PROBLEM: Eating high-calorie foods when offered or when others around you do so.
PLAN: Request help by asking people not to snack around you or offer you food. Encourage them to show you attention in non-food ways.

PROBLEM: Compulsive overeating by always cleaning plate.
PLAN: Always leave some food. Overcome childhood memories of parental approval that required eating all food on our plates. Stop eating when you are full, not when you are stuffed.

PROBLEM: Eating too quickly to realize eating gratification.
PLAN: Make time in your schedule for eating. Use utensils and cut food into smaller pieces. Put fork down between bites and do not reload it until you have finished chewing. Chew slower and more times per mouthful. Get up and take a break during the meal. Consider chopsticks to reduce eating speed.

PROBLEM: Purchasing high-calorie foods.
PLAN: Formulate meals ahead of time so that you may shop from a list to help prevent impulse buying. Don't shop with children and only use coupons for items really needed.

PROBLEM: Eating high-calorie snacks between meals or in certain places.
PLAN: Integrate snacks into your day but plan what and when they will be. Keep to the *eating place* strategy and only eat there (preferably at set times).

"...making gradual substitutions and lifestyle changes."

PROBLEM: Feeling guilty about eating high-calorie food and then eating more.
PLAN: Tell yourself that you are making gradual substitutions and lifestyle changes. There are no forbidden foods but quantities and frequencies should be adjusted. Weight will be lost if you persevere.

PROBLEM: Exercising infrequently.
PLAN: Increase activities of daily living, e.g. keep moving during the day and find ways to increase energy expenditure.

PROBLEM: Trying to short-cut the guidelines of this program.
PLAN: Don't neglect self-monitoring (food and activity diary), consume calories earlier in the day, reduce fat intake, become more active, and get adequate fluid intake. [If you are utilizing this book as part of a monitored weight management program, keep your scheduled office visits.]

PROBLEM: Relying on medication to make you lose weight.
PLAN: Realize that medication is only a tool to assist in controlling appetite and supplement dietary intake while you are changing habits and lifestyle through nutrition education and behavior modification.

"Replace the concept of ideal weight..."

PROBLEM: Unrealistic goal weight.
PLAN: Replace the concept of *ideal weight* with that of clinically significant weight reduction. This is a weight that reduces risk factors without increasing risk of morbidity and mortality. Top fashion models are not realistic weight models for most Americans and may actually be bordering on serious medical problems, including eating disorders.

PROBLEM: Temporary motivation = Temporary weight management.
PLAN: Positive behavior and eating changes incorporated methodically = Permanent weight management tools.

Overeating factors

Overeating can be defined in numerous ways. It can mean too many calories or too much fat intake. It may also mean an exceptionally large single meal or frequent snacking between meals. For the purposes of this book, I will define it to mean excessive intake for an individual's expenditure resulting in excessive, undesired weight. It is important to be aware of overeating since those who have lost and gained weight over and over tend to develop preferences for the sweetest and fattiest foods, eventually leading to more overeating. (For information regarding *Compulsive Overeating*, see page 34.)

Reasons for such inappropriate intake might include the following:

- **Inability to say 'no'** to anything we really want.
- **Meal-times** may be **haphazard** and sometimes **skipped** altogether.
- Due to **poor** dietary education or **motivation**, we consume too many calories and not enough nutrients.
- **Psychological crutch.** Food used for comfort, serenity or relief from boredom or despondency. Binge eating may be a means of anxiety, hostility, or depression release.

Emotions

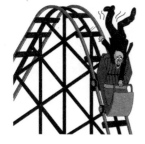

Emotions are just some of the influences upon our eating and lifestyle. They can run the gambit from anger to anxiety, doldrums to depression, or happiness to hostility. Many individuals gain weight because they eat even when their bodies are not signaling hunger. We need to be acutely aware when emotions lie at the root of an overeating problem. Deciding if you're hungry is like deciding if you're in love; if you don't know for sure, you're probably not.

Our emotions can be powerful triggers for eating since they can frequently override what our body is telling us. Many Americans are overweight today as a result of eating in response to emotions.

Boredom is a classic example of an emotional eating cue. Raiding the refrigerator becomes a temporary fix to their boredom. Of course, once the food is gone, the boredom comes back and may leave the person feeling worse for using food as a quick fix. This may then lead to getting more food to soothe the negative feelings they are experiencing and an unhealthy *food-based* circle is established.

Another common emotion people try to solve with food is *depression*. As with boredom, eating temporarily alleviates the depression. Food helps the person escape the unpleasant feeling of depression. Yet, the depression returns when the food is gone and a similar vicious circle is set up, with the person getting even more depressed because of the increasing weight and the apparent lack of self-control.

Food can also serve as a temporary tranquilizer for those who are *anxious* or *nervous*. On and on the list could go. However, the answer for all of these emotional situations is to find alternative ways of dealing with these feelings. Since each person is different, they must find what works best for them (other than food). Hobbies might help with boredom. Counseling or being able to just talk to someone might improve depression. Tension might be alleviated with exercise.

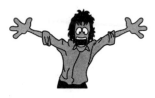

"A food-mood diary will help..."

A *food-mood diary* will help to determine emotional eating. This is similar to a regular food intake journal except you also ask yourself as you are eating, "How do I feel right this minute?" If you are happy, sad, depressed, or anxious, record that feeling next to the food and the time and place it occurred. As you keep these records, look for emotional situations, patterns and triggers to snacking and eating. Begin planning what to do as alternatives to such feelings in the future. Gradually begin to implement these other activities in place of food.

> **FICTION:** One of the best ways to lose weight is to follow a good reducing diet menu whenever you gain weight.
> **FACT:** The best way is to learn how to handle the *conditions* in life that led to the excessive intake in the first place, such as banquets and cocktail parties or emotional upsets. This way you always remain in control over your weight and it never gets away from you.

Hormones

This section will not mention all hormones or try to delve into all aspects of any particular one. It is meant to give a very brief overview and include some considerations that should be mentioned.

Women who physically mature at an early age have a higher tendency towards being more obese. One study shows that by age 30, early maturers had 30 percent more fat than average or late maturers. This points to hormones influencing this excess fat.

Fat tissue is a significant source of *estrogen* produced outside the ovaries. This leads to obese women having higher levels of circulating estrogens than lean women. They also seem to produce a stronger form of estrogen. This may manifest itself as heightened fertility.

"...hormone level may also increase food cravings..."

The increased estrogen hormone level may also increase food cravings in susceptible women. In fact, studies show that an average female typically wants to consume about 150 calories more a day (with a larger percentage being high-carbohydrate foods) as her menstrual period approaches. Tips to help counter these cravings include consuming smaller meals more frequently, increasing non-food related activities, and consuming some type of starch (potato, pasta, rice, or bread) at each meal.

During the last ten days of the menstrual cycle circulating *progesterone* levels are significantly higher than earlier in the cycle. It is during this latter part of the cycle that some women notice cravings for sweets and high-fat foods. This may explain why you have that huge chocolate or sweet craving the week before your cycle starts.

What happens after a complete hysterectomy or menopause? Your doctor may be concerned about osteoporosis or your symptoms may dictate oral estrogen replacement therapy. This is a matter that should be discussed thoroughly with your family doctor. Some women on estrogen therapy seem more likely to develop ovarian and uterine cancer. They may also have increased rates of hypertension, diabetes, pulmonary embolism, and gallbladder disease.

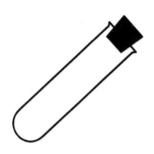

The addition of progesterone to estrogen treatment also has drawbacks. It may increase the rate of heart disease by lowering HDL (good; protective) cholesterol. It can also increase the risk of breast cancer.

"...research continues into hormonal effects..."

To be effective against osteoporosis, estrogen therapy must be continued indefinitely. Some sources state that a woman who has been on estrogen replacement and then stops it is no better off (in terms of bone strength) than if she had not begun the therapy. Other sources think osteoporosis can be slowed if the person's diet is low in animal protein and they get plenty of exercise.

Both *growth hormone* and *thyroid hormone* also play a role in weight, metabolism, and other bodily functions. Over the years, they have been studied extensively and may provide interesting reading. Your own physician should be able to provide you with further information regarding hormones and their influence on your weight.

Even as this is being written, research continues into hormonal effects upon individuals and their weight. One promising field deals with mapping **circadian** (daily) rhythms of various hormones and their effect upon fat cell storage and fat breakdown, something which could lead to entirely new ways of treating obesity and excess weight. We are literally at the edge of a new frontier in our understanding of weight and weight management.

Considerations

Incentives

Lower blood pressure, nicer appearance, better work endurance, or less orthopedic problems may be reward enough for some to make a change in lifestyle, behavior, and eating patterns. Others need some sort of tangible, additional *reward* system.

This is an area where you can be as creative as your imagination will let you. Since you know best what motivates you, look there first. Of course, concentrate on *non-food* related motivators. If new clothes, new shoes, or even just new socks appeal to you, set these as rewards and get them when you reach your *reward trigger*. For rewards for exceptional accomplishments, you might consider things like a movie, good book, ballet, opera, flowers, weekend mini-vacation, or special evening getaway.

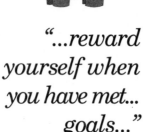

"...reward yourself when you have met... goals..."

You may also make a special bank or savings jar for money you have saved by cutting down on inappropriate foods (especially junk or snack foods). You set the amount—fifty cents to five dollars. It may be helpful if you identify the item(s) you would like and write it on the side of the bank. Once you have accumulated enough money in your *incentive jar* you can buy the desired item.

I would recommend that you reward yourself when you have met behavioral or lifestyle change goals and/or have maintained them fairly consistently for a certain period of time. By using this as an endpoint rather than a certain *weight*, you are focusing on the appropriate areas of weight management.

Self-Esteem

How we really feel about ourselves affects whatever we achieve in life. Perhaps the most important first step in any weight reduction program is building self-esteem. If we improve our self-esteem, this can boost motivation to control our weight. It will also help us to adopt a more positive and brighter outlook on life.

"Parts of self-esteem are attitudes..."

Parts of self-esteem are *attitudes* we have towards ourselves. Since this can influence people's behavior toward nutrition, it is not surprising that anorectic and obese individuals have distorted body images. It has been noticed that women with positive self-esteem consume *better quality* diets than women with poor self-esteem.

One study looked at 153 single women aged 18 to 35 years, assessing the connection between self-esteem, eating patterns, and nutrient intake. Persons with *liberal* lifestyles tended to have inappropriate intake of nutrients. Those with *traditional* lifestyles had sufficient calcium intake and suitable meal patterns. Persons who knew about nutrition and believed it to be important also had acceptable eating habits and nutrient intake. Conclusions from this study were that self-esteem, nutritional attitudes, and knowledge of nutrition can affect nutrient intake and eating habits in young women.

We have all heard that people view themselves differently than other people see them. When obese individuals are given the opportunity to adjust a television monitor screen to reflect their perceived body size, most of them will overestimate (show themselves fatter on the screen than they really are). Of particular interest is that those who were overweight as children are *five times* more likely to overestimate their body size as an adult—even those no longer obese.

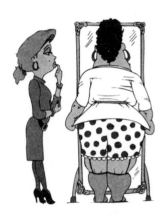

Since body image relates to self-esteem, it is probably best not to be a mirror watcher. As mentioned above, many overweight people cannot accurately assess their body size due to mental distortions. Don't even bother having a family member or friend try to assess your progress. Instead, consider how you feel. Are you experiencing more energy? Do you find yourself less preoccupied with food and hunger?

"...body image relates to self-esteem..."

See the positive things you have been doing for yourself as well. Things such as eating less fat, walking regularly, and being more active in your daily living routine. Realizing your own strengths and weaknesses—and dealing positively with them. Don't forget about how you have been broadening your knowledge of nutrition and healthy habits.

Best of all, you are *staying committed* to a program for life that is dedicated to improving your health, sense of well-being, and proper control of your weight. Realize that you have achieved a lot more than some arbitrary number on the scale.

Goal Setting

This is perhaps one of the most important sections of this book. In order to get someplace or make progress, one has to know where one is going. Whether or not someone has realistic expectations and sets attainable (and desirable) weight reduction goals will determine the long-term success or failure of such effort.

"...you are staying committed to a program for life..."

For numerous years, weight reduction programs have focused on a number on the scale—the so-called *ideal weight*. Attempting to reach it often involved moderate, prolonged caloric restriction and an extremely poor maintenance outcome. 'Scale worship' has probably been a source of failure and frustration for many of you reading this book. We seldom stopped to evaluate what *shape* our bodies were in. If our weight was low enough, we believed ourselves to be thin and healthy. This is reinforced by the fact that the most popular machine at health clubs is the scale.

"Set realistic goals that you can reach..."

Should we throw the scales away? Yes—well almost. Just put them in their proper prospective and use them for self-monitoring on a periodic basis. Recent evidence suggests that achievement of desirable body weight is not the single standard for successful treatment. It doesn't really reflect your physical condition or how fat you are. A healthy weight is one which can be maintained by consuming a nutritious lowfat diet and exercising daily.

What is important? In all reality, very thin looking people can have a lot of fat under their skin or scattered throughout their muscle tissue. Therefore, body fat composition, body mass index and body fat distribution seem to rank high in importance. Your body fat composition is the percentage of body fat compared to lean muscle mass. It should range between 20-26% fat for a woman and 15-22% fat for a man.

Our goals should be oriented towards body fat composition with an eye towards allowing enough time to lose weight safely. Aim for a short term goal of losing 1-2 pounds a week. Initial losses may be more due to associated fluid losses. A long-term goal could be shedding 5 to 15 pounds at a time over a several month period. Tell yourself that several months or more of gradual loss is not unreasonable.

"Forget about past failures."

Set realistic goals that you can reach (like eating fruit in place of doughnuts on your coffee break) instead of unreasonable ones that only lead to disappointment and frustration. Begin by striving for one or two small changes. Some of us would love to lose 40 pounds in one month. Yet, this is unrealistic and dangerous for most of us. Practical goals produce encouraging and long-lasting results. One goal weight could be your lowest weight since age 25 that you maintained for a least one year.

Forget about past failures. Think only of achieving positive results, including improved health, self-esteem, appearance, well-being, energy level, and work performance. Take the time to write out your goals, both long- and short-term. If you need the guidance, even plan out day to day, hour to hour, what to do to meet your goal.

Our suggestion is to change patterns and work on difficult situations, but use whatever you feel appropriate to achieve your goals. Changing dietary selections and lifestyle through substitution and choice is the road to long-term success in weight management. *Lack of sincerity* and *unwillingness to change* are guarantees for failure. This is your life. Don't just be a spectator—participate in it!

One *new focus* of obesity treatment is *medically significant weight loss*. Significant excess body weight, particularly that resulting from excess body fat, begins at levels of 130% to 140% of desirable body weight (body mass index—BMI > 30). By decreasing body weight in 10% to 15% increments, emphasis is on reducing the risk of medical illness, rather than attaining some *ideal* weight. This percentage loss is recommended because it is thought that such controlled weight loss will normalize organ function in 9 out of 10 patients, especially in patients with a body mass index (BMI) greater than 30. In fact, for someone needing to lose fifty pounds, losing just 1/3 of this amount allows them to receive almost 75 percent of the health benefits of losing all fifty.

Obesity-aggravated conditions such as diabetes, hypertension, cardiovascular disease, gallbladder disease and certain cancers could be reduced in some groups. In some studies, a weight loss of 5% of body weight improved some cardiovascular conditions; 10% loss improved some diabetic and hypertensive conditions. Recommendations as to what time frame in which to accomplish this significant weight loss vary, with some extending up to 18 months.

"...lower body fat... lower health risk than abdominal fat..."

Some recommendations call for a period of maintenance of the new body weight for at least six months *before* attempting additional weight reduction (on the order of another 10% to 15%). In short, serial dietary intervention (at yearly intervals) with a short-term goal of reducing body weight 10% to 15% at any intervention and a long-term goal of achieving a BMI < 30 is advocated. This is felt [by those advocating this philosophy] to be a realistic and meaningful short-term goal.

In regards to body fat distribution, *lower body* (gynoid; hip-thigh; 'pear shape') fat distribution represents a lower health risk than *abdominal* (android; truncal; central; 'apple shape') fat patterning. Women tend to have lower body fat patterning, which tends to be harder to lose than man's typical abdominal fat. Fat cells in the hip and thigh area may have higher activity of fat-producing enzymes and mobilize (break-down) fat less effectively than those in the abdomen. Apparently all fat cells are not created equal!

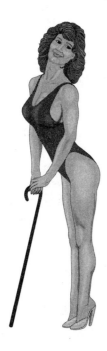

In summary, weight management must be long-term (lifelong) and not oriented to a *goal weight*. We must focus on:
- Control, not a magical cure.
- Maintenance of loss.
- Prevention of gain.
- Realizing the value of modest weight loss (10% or so) as a realistic endpoint.

Realistic expectations

Weight obsession is closely linked to a growing *epidemic* of eating disorders, including anorexia, bulimia, and bingeing. Nothing can be more detrimental physically or mentally than unrealistic expectations and goals.

As a society, we must abandon our current role-models for the *ideal man or woman*. A thirty year survey (1959-1988) of Miss America contestants and Playboy magazine centerfold girls showed a strong trend towards increasing thinness year by year. Currently they are now at anorectic levels of 13 to 19 percent *below* their expected weight. Even average fashion models are about 16 percent underweight. Researchers speculate that weights have leveled off as low as they can be—any lower would risk death!

"...weight control is a lifetime project."

Realize that weight control is a *lifetime* project. The conflict will not be lost or won over a few weeks or months. Patience and stability usually win out. It is not unusual for people who regain lost weight to feel disappointed, disgusted, and ashamed. Many times these negative psychological feelings make it hard to continue seeking the help of health professionals or friends in their weight control efforts.

Change your expectations to wellness solutions, not just weight loss. You can feel good about yourself, eat well in a natural and relaxed way, and enjoy the benefits of being just a little more active than you may currently be. Without the *pressure to perform* you can be more in tune with your internal signals and how true hunger presents itself.

Weight Fluctuations

Body weight fluctuates. Misconception of weight changes can be very frustrating to those attempting to reduce weight. Changes on the scale rarely reflect *only* fatty tissue change. Morning to evening or day to day fluctuations are mainly the result of changes in body fluid and water levels. These, in turn, can be influenced by exercise, hormones (menstrual period), sodium intake, carbohydrates ingested, or fluid consumed.

Weight difference over several weeks tends to reveal changes in levels of fat, muscle and fluids. The scale cannot differentiate what weight loss belongs to which group.

"Too frequent weighing can be confusing..."

Because of this dilemma, some people only weigh once or twice weekly to monitor general *trends*, which is a good recommendation. However, others like to monitor weight daily as a consistent reminder that weight management is a daily event requiring daily attention. Use whatever frequency of weighing that helps you make the lifestyle changes we talk about throughout this book.

No matter how frequently you weigh, try to do so at the same time of day, using the same scale, and clothed similarly. Most people find that the first morning weight, naked or in light bedclothes, and after urination is the best gauge to monitoring progress. If you do not have an accurate or reliable set of scales, remember that some health food stores, pharmacies, and grocery stores maintain pay electronic scales in their store.

Letting your conscience be your guide is probably better than letting the scale do the same. Too frequent weighing can be confusing and play *mind games* with you. If you have appropriate and consistent behavior, your weight will take care of itself.

Over the long-term the scale will not lie. However, weighing daily or more often can lead to several unwanted results. Depression and discouragement can set in if you feel you are doing everything *right* but the scale shows little or no improvement (due to hormone changes, building muscle, fluid shifts, etc.). We may also get the wrong message if we *cheat* and still show weight loss. This gives our subconscious the message that "it's all right to splurge because we can get away with it."

Another time the scale can baffle us is when it goes upward as we start exercise, especially weight training or aerobics, along with a lowfat diet. This can happen as we build lean muscle mass. As we replace the fat in our bodies with muscle, our weight might go up a few pounds at first, but don't let this discourage you. It is only temporary and before long you start to lose the real fat.

Realize that muscle doesn't weigh more than fat. A pound of each weighs the same. However, pound for pound, muscle occupies less *space* than fat so you may notice *inches* being lost more than *pounds*.

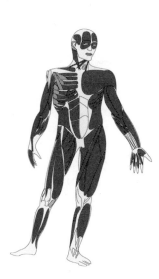

"...muscle doesn't weigh more than fat."

As you reduce fat cell size with weight loss, your body may fill the excess space with fluid, especially if you are a middle-aged woman (or older). This fluid has weight and may sometimes explain why you don't see expected weight loss, even with proper eating and behavioral changes. Physical activity and salt restriction may reduce this water retention.

More and more attention is being directed towards *weight cycling*. This pertains to the typical 'gain-the-weight', followed by the 'lose-the-weight' cycle that most dieters go through. Risks for doing this are being noticed at all weight categories, whether thin or obese.

In a 32-year analysis of weight fluctuations in the Framingham Heart Study, people with high weight variability were 25 to 100 percent more likely to be victims of heart disease and premature death than those whose weight remained stable. Men who gain and lose large amounts of weight in middle adulthood may have a 26 percent increased risk of death from coronary heart disease after age 40. Risk for those in the weight cycling group remained twice as high as for those who experienced no change.

The majority of studies imply that weight cycling does not show negative (undesired) effects on *amount* of total body fat or its *distribution*. It also doesn't seem to cause long-term lowering of resting energy expenditure (basal metabolism). However, as mentioned above, studies do suggest adverse effects through risks of cardiovascular disease and all-cause mortality.

Weight Gain

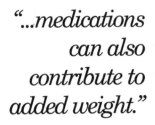

Weight cycling is known to present increased risks in some people. However, don't go to the opposite extreme and purposely gain weight. While some advisors would not recommend weight reduction for some people, no one seems to mind trying *not to gain* unnecessary extra weight throughout our lifetime. In the 30-year Framingham study, no evidence was seen that *weight gains* during middle age increased longevity (life span).

We do know that many things can lead to increased weight. People who eat a lot of high-fat items (typical American diet) may place a large percentage of those calories into their fat cells. Watching this particular area of our intake can often times be of benefit.

Our activity level tends to decrease with age. We go from playing active games as children and getting up and down to change television channels to having our own kids bring us the remote control as we prop our feet up. Being a *desk jockey* at work may also contribute to the dilemma. Age may bring on more illness, which in turn may further limit activity and so on.

"...medications can also contribute to added weight."

Hormonal changes have already been mentioned in another section. Premenstrual cravings for sweets or salty items can certainly add up to weight gain if not modified or controlled. Oral hormone replacement can also have the same effect.

Certain medications can also contribute to added weight. Typical classes of the offending culprits include some types of antidepressants, hormones, anti-inflammatory agents (including steroids), contraceptives, and tranquilizers.

Each year, an average American:

- eats out at restaurants 192 times, including 24 times at McDonald's
- drinks 136.6 gallons of beverages
- drinks 748 cups of coffee
- eats 1460 pounds of food
- eats 244 eggs, including 83 scrambled, 75 fried, 56 boiled, 10 omelets, and 7 poached
- eats 243 bowls of cereal
- eats 24 pounds of cheese, including 10 lbs of cheddar, 5 lbs of mozzarella, 2 lbs of American, and 1 lb of Swiss
- eats 115 pounds of red meat, including 68 lbs of beef, 44 lbs of pork, and 1 lb of lamb & mutton
- eats 57 pounds of poultry, including 44 lbs of chicken & 12 lbs turkey

Mind Games

At one time or another, we have all fallen victim to psychological mind games. Sometimes others influence us, but we are usually our own worst enemy. This is especially true when we can't accept being overweight and continually plan our lives around the day we'll be thin.

We must take personal responsibility for our own eating behavior. It is imperative that psychological barriers to weight control are identified and overcome. They are the very heart of most weight control problems. We can then use the power of our mind in a positive and productive way.

As part of weight management, we can draw from a part of medicine which has focused on what is called *Cognitive Behavior Therapy*. This is a fancy name for our bringing awareness of our thoughts and perceptions into our conscious spotlight, including understanding and reasoning.

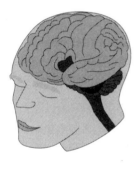

If this still sounds like Greek to you, look at improper behavior and eating patterns as stemming from a three-fold process. The first is *irrational beliefs and fears* which in turn lead to *negative emotional states*. The irrational beliefs come from the difference between the belief and the reality of whether something can or cannot be done. Irrational ones ultimately lead to *out of control* behaviors (such as bingeing), which reinforces the irrational beliefs and the process continues to build. Just as one link of a chain is tied into the other, so are these processes.

"...irrational beliefs or thoughts can be very damaging."

In order to break this detrimental cycle and treat it effectively, therapy has to begin at the first link in the chain, **irrational beliefs**. Effective therapy has to be somewhat like a good trial lawyer. First, the evidence at the base of these irrational thoughts must be examined. Next, these thoughts must be challenged as being irrational. Finally, you must offer the jury a different explanation of the situation, or in this *case* reinforce alternative thoughts and actions based upon appropriate, rational, good health and nutrition principles.

You should probably write down some of your own personal thoughts. By doing so, you crystallize the intangible and make yourself consciously aware of them. Some of the irrational ones you may find could be similar to the following:

- **"crystal ball gazing"**— It occurred this way in the past and it will occur this way again. Last time I ate one french fry I couldn't stop, so it will probably happen the next time I eat one.
- **"shifting the blame"**— Foods with refined sugar or white flour *always* make me hungry and lose control.
- **"all-or-none"** rule — Once I start the package, I always finish it. If I blow one meal, I might as well blow the rest of the day and start fresh tomorrow (or Monday).

These underlying irrational beliefs or thoughts can be very damaging. They are often accompanied by either a deep fear of weight gain or a distorted body image. Deep fear can cause irrational thoughts similar to those that follow:

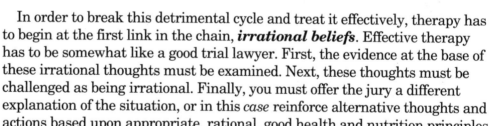

"Eating *always* leads to loss of self-control. Once it begins, I can't stop it. The result is brief discomfort and long-term obesity. The solution (*though irrational*) is (1) not to eat anything I like or not eat at all, or (2) eat when and what I want, bingeing if I so desire, and then starve or purge later."

Distorted body image manifests itself by our perception of what is *normal* and what constitutes being *fat*. This can sometimes be hard to readjust.

"...the feeling of being out of control."

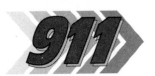

The next link in our cognitive behavioral chain is the **negative emotions** that result from the irrational thoughts. If you inwardly believe you cannot succeed you will be unable to succeed. Given these previous thought patterns, any eating encounter is begun with fear and reluctance. Eating then leads to panic or depression (for not being *good*). These feelings of fear or panic then confirm the feeling of being out of control. This reinforces the feeling of losing control, which can lead to even more bingeing.

We must realize that past failures do not prevent future successes. Yet, once we crash into the *out of control* feeling, we figuratively call '911' and go into typical *emergency protocols*. These may include:
- renewed resolve to shun what we consider to be forbidden foods (e.g. sugar, caffeine, white flour, etc.) — all or none behavior.
- hopelessness and self-disgust — depression.
- purging or laxative abuse — neutralizing behavior.
- determination to maintain firmer control over eating — restricted eating.

If you have ever experienced any of these thoughts or patterns, you can appreciate why it becomes so important to identify these irrational thoughts and fears and confront and change them in a logical and appropriate manner. Reinforcement of new attitudes and behaviors may take awhile, but the time and energy is well spent.

The remainder of this section will cover thoughts, beliefs, and attitudes with pertinent comments about them. I hope identifying them and putting them in a fresh light will assist you in your own changes.

I'll succeed if I only eat one meal a day. Many weight-reducers are led to the weight counselor's office out of desperation. They cannot figure out why they stay heavy only eating once a day. If they are prone to slow metabolism or have been doing this off and on as part of a long-standing gain-lose cycle, this can backfire. The body's metabolism can go into *emergency* conservation (starvation mode) whereby calories that are consumed are stored with extreme efficiency. In these cases, as little as 2000 to 2500 calories may produce a pound of fat, instead of the usually quoted 3500 calories needed to gain a pound. To counter this starvation mode, spread the 900 to 1000 calories consumed daily during weight reduction over three, four or five moderately-spaced feedings.

"I have to be perfect..."

I have to be perfect on my diet. Certain individuals truly believe that their eating behavior has to be perfect. The problem with this is that it sets a sure course for failure. Such people are always striving to do better instead of being proud of what benefits they have accomplished. They'll complain about missing their self imposed goal by a half pound rather than seeing the progress they are making. These are the type that tend to give up on dieting because it is too hard (actually it's impossible under their standards).

Just this once ... Some people play the game of modifying their behavior and eating patterns except on weekends, while traveling, when dining out, on vacation, at banquets or birthday celebrations, or the weekly bridge club meeting. One or two major exceptions a week can cancel five to six days of superb self-discipline and commitment. Adding all of the *just once* occasions can make for frequent diversions from the path you have chosen.

Feast or famine. This all-or-nothing attitude towards weight control often weakens a successful program. A typical scenario may show someone following healthy behavioral and eating patterns for several weeks. However, the co-workers at the office want her to join them for Mexican food at lunch. She goes and helps herself to some of the appealing nacho appetizers, even before she really thinks about it. Her reasoning may then justify that "since she has blown her diet anyway, anything is fair game." The 3200 calorie meal that follows and the overindulging the remainder of the week tends to be a behavioral disaster. Following a sensible program even at a 75 percent level is better than zero percent. A better alternative is to abandon all-or-none thinking and realize eating lapses will occur. Nobody is perfect and they can learn from their mistakes, if they really want to.

I can't succeed at anything. When people don't succeed at something, particularly weight reduction, they often start developing feelings of failure. Simply faltering in a weight program does not make you a failure. Always remember, *to falter is not to fail*. The only way someone can truly be a failure in weight management is to give up entirely. If you don't expect to be successful, you won't be. If you constantly tell yourself you have no willpower, you won't have any. Like your muscles, willpower has to be exercised in order to strengthen it. Remember Thomas Edison, the inventor of the lightbulb? After several thousand unsuccessful attempts at developing it, he was asked, "After so many unsuccessful attempts at this, don't you feel you have been a failure?" His answer should inspire us all. His reply, "No, indeed I do not. I now know several thousand things that *won't* work."

"...to falter is not to fail."

I can do this by myself. We sometimes feel that excess weight is a character flaw or an admission of weakness. Our pride gets in the way and we feel we can conquer this problem if we just keep our mouths shut and go exercise. While some independence is important in weight management, of equal importance is being open minded and receptive to expert advice. Well known professional golfers and baseball players frequently have a personal coach that may travel with them. They *constantly* work on proper hand placement, stance, proper timing, etc. Even physicians and dietitians with weight problems can benefit by advice and management by another professional.

I need to lose weight quickly. One aspect of weight management that is highly over-rated is the *rate* of weight loss. No studies support the idea that *faster* weight loss is *better*. In fact, results would seem to indicate the opposite is true. Don't forget the story of the tortoise and the hare and who won in the long-run. In evaluating weight management programs, one should be more concerned with safety of the program, whether weight lost is fat, muscle, or fluid, and long-term success rates of the participants.

"...you have under-taken diets improperly..."

Weight management is too difficult. Our natural inclination is to take the path of least resistance and give up anything challenging even before we start it. We typically want to be *spoon-fed* what to eat, when to eat it, and not have to be bothered with being responsible for ourselves, our actions, and our eating behavior. The wise person realizes this and takes the attitude that while something may be difficult, at least initially, it is not impossible and it *certainly* is worthwhile.

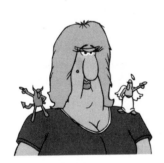

I've been bad this week. You have to get away from the *good cop—bad cop* scenario. Realize that you have a goal, and that goal is to manage your weight and be healthy. Things you do will either be *appropriate* or *inappropriate* towards reaching your goal. Doing inappropriate things doesn't make you a good or bad person, it just delays your time frame. To falter is not to fail! Okay, so you made inappropriate choices. It would have been better not to have made them, but it's not the end of the world. The *real* learning experience is realizing what can be done in the future to keep from getting side-tracked over and over again.

I always do badly staying on a diet. Refrain from absolutes like *always, never, must,* and similar thinking. You can be honest with yourself and think 'I *usually* do badly on a diet', but you must realize that you have undertaken diets improperly and without proper guidance in the past. How many math problems in elementary school did you work through before you mastered principles with proper teaching? The same can be said of your undertaking appropriate weight management techniques.

It's not fair. Because of our own unique chemistry and genetics, we may distribute fat differently, have a lower rate of metabolism, or have more trouble with certain types of activities than others. Certainly that's not fair. But just as these factors can be liabilities, our own uniqueness also carries with it our own set of assets. Through hard work and training we can offset these handicaps and overcome our disadvantages. Don't waste another minute in grumbling about your weight problem and its causes. Realize that there are things you can do and get started doing them today.

Poor me—martyrdom. How often do we spend time and energy getting those around us to feel sorry for us because of the *sacrifices* we are making to lose weight? How many of us go on vacation and constantly complain about how much things are costing? Sure, we think of this at times but don't we usually dwell on the enjoyable, positive, and fun aspects of what we are doing? It certainly leaves us wanting another vacation next year, doesn't it? In a similar manner, don't dwell on the price you are paying for success. Instead, look at what you are getting. New found energy, agility, looking and feeling better, more youthful appearance, and the surprised looks of casual contacts that notice the *new you* should be powerful motivators.

> *"Easy come, easy go works in reverse too."*

I'm looking for the shortcut. Like the lost city of Atlantis, most of us have tried to find that mythical *quick-fix* weight program. This dream is perpetuated by unethical quick weight loss advertisements and programs in the media. If such a shortcut existed, I would share it with you. Most quick reducing diets give the illusion of easy weight loss through resulting loss of muscle and fluid, along with some fat. *Easy come, easy go* works in reverse too. This counterfeit weight loss is usually gained back very quickly after the *diet* is over.

Inappropriate goals and expectations. A person may be disillusioned and disappointed in their own eyes for not losing enough weight, even though their physician or nutritionist feels they are doing well. This is because of the hype of our culture and our own *unrealistic goals* based upon that hype. Don't use professional models or Miss America contestants as your weight role-model, most are medically underweight. Perfectionism (allowing no room for error) in weight management has a built-in guarantee of failure. Once you vary from your diet *even slightly*, the diet in your mind is over. Also, contentment with excess weight can be inappropriate too. Attitudes of poor or ethnic groups with high amounts of obesity may view weight loss as the result of a serious illness or decreasing a woman's sexual attractiveness.

I deserve this food and drink. This thought usually comes at the end of a long day or especially stressful and/or grueling situation. The appropriate rebuttal to this line of thinking is that if you continue to use food and drink as a reward, you will either need to exercise more or else will reduce at a slower rate. What you *deserve* is to feel and be the best you can be!

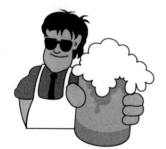

> *"I deserve this food and drink."*

Sabotage and undermining. This can come from a friend, relative, party hostess, or even worse, your spouse. Your new lifestyle may be taking away the thrill of culinary pleasures they are accustomed to. Even more basic is the feelings of a non-reducing (and usually overweight) spouse that you are bettering yourself to be more attractive to others. They may even fear you leaving them for someone else. If reassurance and talking to them about your health and happiness as motivation for weight loss doesn't solve the problem, professional counseling is in order. Spousal competition in losing weight can also discourage the female if she doesn't take into account that a male has about 20% more muscle mass and therefore tends to lose weight faster over any given time period. Males may have the genetic edge, but perseverance wins for you too.

"...toning activity may also improve your figure..."

I don't need exercise. A typical mistake made when undertaking weight reduction is trying to conquer the problem without exercise. Recent studies only verify that long-term success in weight management is highly correlated with maintaining (or starting) some form of exercise. At the very least, increasing your *activities of daily living* should help. Besides weight maintenance, a multitude of other benefits can be gained for some. These include improved lipids (cholesterol, triglycerides), blood sugar, coronary and peripheral circulation, as well as being a great source of stress reduction and natural antidepressant. Proper toning activity may also improve your figure as it tightens and firms areas due to underlying muscle tone.

I don't have time for exercise. The truth is, we have time for anything we *really* consider important. You can find the time if you plan your daily activities wisely. If you had a day in court, jury duty, or had to pick up a two thousand dollar sweepstakes check, you would *make* the time to be in those various places, wouldn't you? Which of these things are *more* important than your health, appearance, and overall sense of well being?

POUND PSALM

Strict is my diet, I must not want.

It maketh me to lie down at night hungry: it leadeth me past Baskin Robbins.

It trieth my willpower: it leadeth me in the paths of starvation for my figure's sake.

Yea, though I walk through the aisles of the pastry department, I will buy no sweet rolls; for they are fattening; the cakes and pies, they tempt me.

Before me is a table with celery and lettuce; my day's quota runneth over.

Surely calories and weight charts shall follow me all the days of my life; and I shall dwell in the fear of the scales forever.

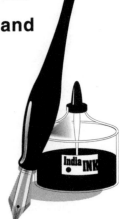

Obesity

Just as there are a multitude of weight treatments, so are there a multitude of definitions for obesity. Obesity, in Latin, means *to eat* and thus does not relate its complex etiology. While no precise medical definition exists, many would agree that it is a condition of excess body fat (or adipose tissue) that may adversely affect health. In some cases, the excess body fat of obesity is independent of weight.

A working definition of *obesity* could be *the condition in which a person carries excessive body fat*. Adult males should carry no more than 15-22% of their total body weight as fat. Adult females should carry no more than 20-26% fat. The average body fat percentage of Americans is 23% for males and 32% for females.

Some practitioners define adiposity (excess body fat) by weight. They use *overweight* to mean 110-119 percent over optimal weight. Overweight then is an increased body weight in relation to height. They define obesity as 120 percent or more over optimal weight. Regardless of the definition used, most overweight adults put on their extra pounds between ages 25 and 35.

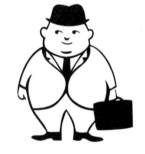

"...*obesity affects about 26% of adult Americans...*"

Body mass index (BMI) has been advocated in the past by some researchers to categorize patients into various health risk categories. The BMI value for obesity (depending upon the researcher) ranges from 27 to 30 or more. Above average mortality rates become apparent at approximately a BMI > 28. Severe obesity is a BMI > 35 and is associated with about twice the increase in total mortality (death) and several times increased risk of death due to a variety of diseases.

Other researchers focus on body fat and the circumference in a waist-to-hip ratio. However, this ratio is a poor measure of visceral fat (inside abdomen) compared to multiscan computed tomography (CT) techniques. Certain health risks are greater depending upon where the fat tissue is actually located (especially in the visceral—abdominal—compartment). Therefore, measurement of this visceral fat volume becomes important.

A new technique of measuring the front-to-back (sagittal) diameter of the abdomen in patients lying on their backs at the level of their upper hip bone (iliac crest) seems to be a very good predictor of the abdominal (visceral) fat volume. Time will tell whether this will replace the use of BMI and waist/hip ratio in future research.

From data gathered in 1976-1980, we find obesity affects about 26 percent (34 million; one in four) of adult Americans age 20 to 74 — considered to be 20% or more above their desirable weight. About 12 million individuals are 40% or more above their ideal weights and are considered severely overweight. Of adolescents age 12 to 19, fifteen percent were classified as obese.

In some populations, particularly minorities, the rates of obesity are much higher — up to three times the rate of white populations. The occurrence for black women is 45 percent, compared with 25 percent for white women. Obesity among black teenagers has increased 53 percent in the past 20 years, compared with a 35 percent increase for white teens.

Are we a nation obsessed with weight? Consider that nearly 90% of Americans think they weigh too much, and more than 35% want to lose 15 pounds or more. At any given time, approximately 50 percent of women and 25 percent of men are trying to lose weight. A Gallup Poll in 1987 reported that 31% of American women, ages 19-39, diet at least once a month. Of that group, 16% saw themselves as perpetual dieters. Dieting attempts seem to be starting younger these days; among high school students, 44 percent of females and 15 percent of males are attempting to lose weight.

"Are we a nation obsessed with weight?"

Many worry about being overweight for obvious social reasons. Their motives to be thin include appearance, attractiveness, and self-esteem. Of equal or greater importance should be a concern for good health. For the time being, obesity is a lifelong but *controllable* disease process.

Attitudes towards obesity and the obese have only recently begun to change. It has only been since 1985 that obesity has been *officially* recognized as a disease. Maddox et al (1968) found that physicians regarded overweight patients as weak willed, ugly, and awkward. In a study of health care professionals, Maimon et al (1979) found that 84% considered the obese to be self-indulgent, 88% assumed they ate to compensate for other problems, and 70% assumed they were emotionally disturbed. A study at a large university several years ago found respondents stating a marriage *preference* for embezzlers, drug addicts, shoplifters, those with poor hygiene, or criminals *over someone overweight*.

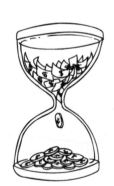

Prejudice against weight is often accompanied by discrimination, even in the workplace. In one report, 16% of employers stated they would not hire obese individuals under any circumstances. An additional 44% said they would hire them only under special conditions.

Health care costs of obesity are estimated at $140 billion dollars per year in direct and indirect costs. This does not include another $30 billion spent annually on commercial weight loss products and programs (not including surgery), and an estimated $5 to $6 billion on fraudulent products. If you add money spent on smoking for weight control (about 1 in 5 women smokers) or mainline cosmetic products for such non-proven uses as *cellulite* treatment, you begin to get a sense of the magnitude of the problem.

"...no single treatment intervention is ideal."

Whatever else can be said about obesity, no single treatment intervention is ideal. None work to perfection but each may contribute to partial

"...prevention of additional gain is needed."

success. Many patients report that sticking to a program of dieting and lifestyle changes gets tougher after the first ten weeks or so. Therefore, we need ways to enhance motivation and interest throughout.

Better management of the weight lost or prevention of additional gain is needed. When hypertensive medications or cholesterol-lowering medications are stopped, those medical problems often return to their pre-treatment state. Therefore, weight regain after treatment *does not* indicate failure. It actually shows the intervention was successful during the treatment.

Obesity Consequences & Risks

Our dietary intake plays a role in atherosclerosis, certain cancers, diabetes mellitus, heart disease, stroke, and obesity. Diet also contributes to osteoporosis and dental diseases.

As mentioned earlier, we will use 20 percent or more above desired body weight to define obesity. This definition covers about one in four adult Americans, or 34 million people. No matter what definition is used, obesity is a common health problem in the U.S.; estimates range from 26-40% of all adults to 15-27% of all children (depending upon the definition used). It has been called one of the most prevalent debilitating chronic diseases in the U.S. It robs the individual of their productiveness and stamina, and the nation of needed health care assets, as potentially billions of health care dollars could be salvaged from unnecessary medical and surgical interventions for obesity associated diseases.

Moderate amounts of body fat do not appear to compromise general health in some studies. Obesity related health risks seem to be associated with overall weight, total body fat, pattern of fat distribution, and *when* the weight was gained. For example, gaining 20 extra pounds during adulthood almost doubles the risk of heart disease. In addition, a study done by the American Cancer Society showed that persons more than 40 percent above average weight showed doubling of the risk of death from coronary heart disease.

Excess upper body and abdominal fat ('apple shape') carries a greater risk of ill-health; e.g. diabetes, heart disease, elevated blood pressure. Individuals with increased intra-abdominal fat are referred to as having central obesity or upper-body or android pattern of fat distribution. Central obesity is associated with metabolic disturbances, hyperinsulinemia and insulin resistance to a greater extent than is lower-body obesity. It is also a strong independent risk factor for cardiovascular disease (morbidity and mortality).

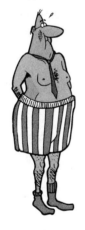

"Central obesity contrasts with lower body... obesity..."

Central obesity contrasts with lower body or gynoid obesity ('pear shape') in which the increase in adipose mass occurs primarily below the

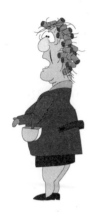

waist. Surplus fat in the buttocks and thighs has relatively minor risks. This lower body (hip-thigh) fat was designed for women as an energy reserve should famine occur during pregnancy or breast-feeding. Fat in this area may be more difficult for women to lose (and perhaps unhealthy to attempt to) because of its inherent design and purpose.

Women within a healthy range (body mass index or percent body fat) may be better off exercising to maintain body shape rather than continually dieting. Accept the circumstances and concentrate on enjoying life. If you are curious about your distribution of fat, the waist-to-hip ratio can be used.

"Risks increase with the degree of obesity."

Aside from dietary intake and fat distribution having consequences, we need to realize other lifestyle habits are important too. A 1979 report by the Surgeon General on Health Promotion and Disease stated that over 50% of deaths, disease and health status change in the U.S. are related to individual *lifestyle health habits*. In plain English, this means that we are directly responsible and can control circumstances leading to over half the deaths in this country.

Risks increase with the *degree* of obesity. In general, they begin to reach importance at a weight greater than 20 percent above optimal, or at a body mass index (BMI) greater than 27. The risk of both non-fatal and fatal coronary disease among women in the heaviest BMI was more than *three times higher* than that in the leanest group.

The appropriate dividing lines for defining obesity may differ for Mexican-Americans. Several studies indicate that they may tolerate higher body weight without increasing the risk of death. Other ethnic populations may need to have their own specifically defined risk points.

The life-span of the average American has increased an extra 40 years over the past century. Instead of dying at an early age of 35 or 40 from famine or infections, we now live longer and succumb to a different group of diseases — diabetes, cancer, high blood pressure, and heart disease. Many of these diseases have a significant (but not exclusive) relationship to obesity. Remarkably, some of the aforementioned diseases can be prevented or treated by eliminating obesity.

"Risks also seem to increase with the duration of obesity..."

Risks also seem to increase with the *duration* of obesity, including childhood-onset obesity. Death rates ranged from 110 percent with an obesity history of 0-5 years, to 169 percent with 15-22 years of obesity. The largest differences were seen for both younger men and women.

Obesity is an independent risk factor for both high blood pressure, as well as for heart disease. Even a *mild to moderate* overweight condition is associated

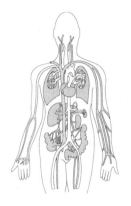

with an 80 percent elevation of coronary risk. Women of average weight had coronary risks approximately 30 percent higher than those of lean women.

Since the blood in an overweight person must be pumped over greater distances (an extra pound needs a mile of blood vessels for nutrient support), blood pressure may increase to make sure the blood will reach the farthest point in the circulatory system. The blood supply to the heart can often be decreased due to this increased workload and higher blood pressure. Not only is the heart made to work harder, it may be forced to do so with less oxygen — a prime set-up for a heart attack.

Obesity Complications and Risks

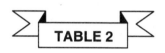

TABLE 2

*atherosclerosis -- injury to arteries, including hardening	blood pressure elevation -- 3x risk vs. normal weight individual	*cancer -- cervix, colon, kidney, ovary, prostate, thyroid. Women > 40% overwt.--5x risk of uterine cancer vs. normal
cholesterol elevation -- 2x risk vs. normal. Also have higher LDL (bad) and low HDL (good) cholesterol.	*diabetes -- 3x more common in obese person. Higher incidence of type II diabetes (non-insulin dependent).	digestive tract disease, including fatty infiltration of the liver (may cause abnormal blood tests)
endocrine imbalance, including menstrual irregularities	gallbladder disease, gallstones	gout and gouty arthritis
*heart disease -- enlarged heart, congestive heart failure, coronary disease	hirsutism -- abnormal hairiness (especially in women)	infertility -- trouble attaining pregnancy or carrying to term
insulin resistance -- hyperinsulinism	longevity decrease (earlier death)	lung disease -- chronic obstructive pulmonary disease, low oxygenation
mobility decrease -- restricted motion or agility	osteoarthritis -- degenerative arthritis (usually hips & knees)	Pickwickian syndrome (poor air exchange and sleepiness due to obesity)
polycystic ovary	pregnancy -- high risk	psychosocial incapacity
salt sensitivity higher	skin hyperpigmentation and infections (fungal and yeast)	sleep apnea (periods of non-breathing)
*stroke (cerebral vascular accident -- CVA)	surgical risks and post-operative complication risks increased	thrombophlebitis and pulmonary embolus risk increase
triglyceride elevation	varicose veins	weight-related injuries

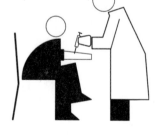

*Five of the ten leading causes of death in the U.S. to which obesity is a major contributor.

"...obesity has adverse effects on health and longevity."

There are several potential things that may *increase* disease and death risks in overweight patients. Some of these are as follows:

- Below normal stature
- Excess visceral (gut) fat
- Impaired health not attributable to overweight
- Obesity of prolonged duration
- Obesity associated risk factors (as in Table 2)

- Ethnic group known to be vulnerable to obesity problems
- Family history premature coronary heart disease, gout, diabetes, hypertension

Table 2 (page 57) is a listing of some of the complications, increased risks, and problems known or highly suspected to be related to excess weight and obesity. They represent dermal, cardiac, digestive, endocrine, obstetric, orthopedic, and pulmonary problems that have been observed. Besides those listed, there may also be adverse social, psychological and economic consequences, which in turn can lead to anxiety, depression and poor self-image. You may wish to use this table for positive re-enforcement of behavioral changes for your weight management.

Obesity and Death

Social reasons motivate many people's concern for obesity. *Good health* would be a better reason since the death rate from all causes increases as weight rises. In 1985 the National Institutes of Health held a consensus conference on the health implications of obesity. The report concludes by stating, "The evidence is now overwhelming that obesity has adverse effects on health and longevity. Obesity is clearly associated with hypertension, hypercholesterolemia, diabetes and excess of certain cancers and other medical problems." The NIH experts agreed that people 20% or more above their ideal body weight are medically at risk. This risk becomes substantial for people who weigh more than 30% above their ideal weight.

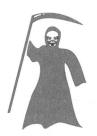

Death rates for *obese males* are higher from accidents, diabetes, kidney disease, stroke, and cancers of the colon, rectum, and prostate. One study showed that men who weighed between 100 and 109 percent of desirable weight had the lowest death rate over thirty years. Other risk surveys show that 15% excess weight leads to a 10% increased mortality compared to average males. Thirty-five percent excess weight has roughly a 35% mortality increase. Males 50% over their ideal weight show over a 70% increase in death rates.

Obese women have higher mortality due to arteriosclerotic kidney disease and cancers of the gallbladder, biliary tract, breast, uterus, and ovaries.

"Is weight loss beneficial?"

Is weight loss beneficial, especially considering that one study showed at 25-fold increase in diabetes mortality among obese young women? The incidence and severity of noninsulin-dependent diabetes mellitus and hypertension in overweight persons are reduced by weight loss. Reducing also affects risk factors for cardiovascular disease, improving lipid and lipoprotein levels. Among very obese individuals, weight loss has been followed by greater functional status, reduced work absenteeism, less pain, and greater social interaction. The prevalence and severity of sleep apnea also can be substantially reduced by weight reduction.

Although there seems to be little doubt that overweight individuals have increased risk for morbidity and mortality, it does not immediately follow that weight loss reduces that increased risk. Further consideration of what weight, if any, should be lost should be discussed with a person's family physician and based upon sound health principles.

Table 3, adapted from the 1979 Build & Blood Pressure Study shows increased mortality with rise in weight for insured men and women:

TABLE 3

If you are above average weight by:	Your chance of death compared to normal is:	
	for men	for women
10%	11% higher	6% higher
20%	20%	10%
30%	33%	25%
40%	50%	36%
50%	71%	???

[In this Build Study, increase in mortality with excess weight is steeper in young adults (ages 20-49) than for older men and women (ages 50-69).]

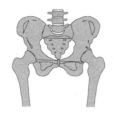

For those electing to maintain excess weight, there may be one health benefit you may be interested in. Obesity may help a woman slow down osteoporosis and keep her bone mass density at more optimum levels. Osteoporotic hip fracture appears to be less common in obese women. The reason for this is theorized to be due to the bone keeping more mass to support the extra weight during the adult years.

Causes of Obesity

The causes of obesity are not well understood, but research with animals and humans suggest many factors, many of them complex. A listing could include interrelation among genetics, environment, psychological and social factors, metabolic components, physical inactivity, high-fat dietary intake, and behavioral influences. Small increases in percent body fat can occur without increasing body weight, and overweight can occur in the absence of increased caloric intake.

"...obesity may be a relatively recent problem."

It seems that obesity may be a relatively recent problem. Early primitive people were generally hunting and gathering societies. There are *no* reported cases of obesity among people who used hunting and gathering as their way of life. Obesity has become a threatening and pervasive health problem in only select societies—those distinguished by affluence, economic modernization, food surplus, and social stratification.

Our environment of readily available, highly palatable high-fat foods is but one of several factors causing obesity. It is these tasty foods high in fat and calorically dense that promote overconsumption and therefore encourage obesity in vulnerable individuals. Unfortunately, large fat stores do not slow down this overconsumption and biological drive to eat.

It has even been noted that transient food deprivation in a pregnant mother can lead to adult obesity in her child. The body has a strong defense against undernutrition and only a minimal response to the effects of overnutrition. Recent research also suggests a diurnal (daily) fluctuation of certain hormones causing a shift toward either fat storage or fat breakdown, depending upon high and low hormone times and their phases (time relationship).

Affluent cultures (e.g. United States) have made physical exercise a commodity. Decades ago, people would come home and *rest* after their workday. Now they come home after 'work' and *exercise*. Today we burn energy through daily workouts rather than daily work.

Scientists have looked at obesity in terms of whether fat cell *number* or fat cell *size* (weight) increase in adult obesity. Our current understanding is that fat cell size increases up to about 66 pounds of body fat, while fat cell number increases over the whole body fat range. Therefore, *moderate* obesity is usually due to enlarged individual fat cell size. *Severe* obesity is usually due to increased number of fat cells (or a combination of size *and* number).

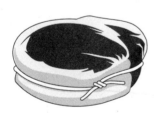

If you are overweight, it's probably not because you eat too much *food* but too much *fat*. Several studies have shown that overweight people often do not eat more than normal weight individuals. The body fat we store comes mainly from food we consume. It has been estimated that between 97 to 98% of fat we eat is *never* used for energy by our bodies, but goes into our fat cells instead. Fat production by our liver is only a minor contributor to overall fat production. Daily breakdown of fat from the fat cells is low (slow) in obese patients who have lost weight and doesn't increase with fat intake.

The activity of an important *fat-producing* enzyme, lipoprotein lipase (LPL), has been found to be defective in certain individual's muscle and fat tissue. In obese and those who were obese but have lost weight, this enzyme's (LPL) activity is increased in fat tissue in both the fasting state (period of not eating) and after eating carbohydrates. Therefore, it seems to encourage fat production in these individuals.

You don't have to be a world-class gymnast or marathon runner to prevent excess weight. Just become more active than you currently are. Some may find aerobic exercise helpful but such recommendations must come from your physician after a thorough evaluation of your health, lifestyle, and personal physical limitations.

Metabolism

"Basal metabolic rate is about 50-70% of daily energy use."

Daily energy use can be divided into three main parts: resting (basal) metabolic rate, the thermic (heat-producing) effect of food, and energy used by physical activity. The resting skeletal muscle metabolism seems to be a major component of the whole-body metabolism. Basal metabolic rate is about 50-70% of daily energy use. The thermic effect of food represents another 10%, while physical activity (in sedentary adults) utilizes the remaining 20-40% of daily energy expenditure. The energy cost of any activity is higher in the obese, although sometimes they may have lower activity levels. Of interest is that some studies have shown obese subjects having higher metabolic rates than lean subjects.

Our definition of metabolism will be 'the transformation by which energy is made available for various uses by the body'. *Basal metabolism* is the minimal energy used for the maintenance of respiration, circulation, bowel activity, muscle tone, body temperature, glandular activity, and the other low-level functions of the body. Whether our body burns energy (calories) like a candle or a bonfire depends on multiple factors, including body lean and fat mass, age, sex, genetics, activity, food, and hormones.

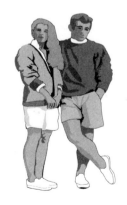

A man's basal metabolism (resting energy level) is about 7% higher than a woman's due to his larger ratio of muscle-to-fat. Since muscle is one of the largest calorie-burning parts of the body, even at identical heights and weights, men burn more calories than women. This is why you should refrain from comparing your weight-loss to your spouse.

With every decade of age past your thirtieth birthday, maintenance calorie requirements drop by about 2 to 8 percent, depending upon the individual. If at forty you still eat like you did at age twenty, don't be puzzled by the bulges. Unless you're exceptionally active, you'll have to cut back as you get older *just to stay even*. If that doesn't sound appealing, realize that resting energy needs may vary by 30% or more for persons of the same age and sex. This continues to point out the individual variations among us all.

"...men burn more calories than women."

Since our bodies try to fight undernutrition, when we purposely reduce calories beyond a certain level our own metabolic rate can fall. Within 24 to 48 hours after caloric restriction begins, a person's resting metabolic rate can drop. This drop can exceed 20% in as little as 2 weeks and may exert marked influence on body weight.

One study showed that when experimental rats lost 14.9% of their weight by restriction of calories, their resting metabolism dropped by 24.6%. Another report showed that obese patients undergoing weight reduction dropped their daily maintenance requirement by 28%.

Whether adding a physical training program during weight reduction can protect against the fall in basal metabolism is controversial. It is known that exercise-trained individuals have a higher resting metabolic rate than nontrained ones.

Future of Weight Management

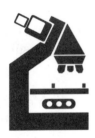

Research continues into the physiologic mechanisms of obesity and excess weight. Several mechanisms of excess weight have been targeted for potential therapeutic intervention. Some of the areas under study include stimulation of fat breakdown, increasing body heat production (metabolic), slowing or inhibiting stomach emptying, new appetite suppressants, blocking carbohydrate or fat digestion, and manipulation of diurnal (daily) hormonal cycles to reduce susceptibility of the body's fat cells for fat storage.

Certain substances, called peptides, have been found to increase or reduce an individual's preferences for certain nutrients in the diet. It may be possible to give *select* peptides to someone and have them *reduce* their craving for fat or simple sugars. Others peptides may *increase* protein desires. Combinations of many effects are theoretically possible.

"...anorexants mainly work on appetite..."

Newer and safer appetite suppressants continue to be sought. As scientists learn more about the brain and neurotransmitters, exciting thresholds lie within reach, just waiting to be broken. Remember though, anorexants mainly work on appetite and *do not* change inappropriate eating behavior, cause a reduction in fat intake, or make a person more active.

Circadian-rhythm based weight management may hold promise for the future. This involves mapping and changing certain physiologic hormone levels and their daily highs and lows, which may influence fat cells' ability to store fat. Imagine being able to eat almost anything you want and not having all the excess calories packed away into the fat cells. Sound too good to be true? Stay tuned...

General Health

It has become apparent that the origins of obesity that contribute to so many of today's health problems have a firm basis in our diets so heavily laden with fat. Of equal importance would also be our gravitation to sedentary lifestyles.

Since it has been said that the field of medicine can only influence about 15-20% of our health complications, we can view with excitement the revelation that we can *prevent or abolish* most of these diseases by adopting healthier lifestyles of eating and exercise. This is what weight management really is; a component of overall health management.

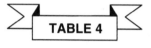

TABLE 4

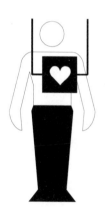

Proportional (%) Contributions to Premature Death (Estimates)			
Disease	**Lifestyle**	**Heredity**	**Health Services**
Cancer	61	29	10
Diabetes	34	60	6
Heart Disease	63	25	12
Liver Disease	79	18	3
Stroke	72	21	7
AVERAGE	61.8	30.6	7.6

Chart adapted from 1982 Stanford Heart Disease Prevention Program

Armed with the knowledge that excess weight can cause high blood pressure (the *silent killer*), and knowing that persons with hypertension have three to four times the normal risk of developing coronary heart disease, it is certainly motivating to do what we can to prevent acquiring high blood pressure. And of course, no one wants the seven times increased risk of stroke that hypertension can bring.

Besides controlling weight and some of the associated risk factors just mentioned, watching our diets may also be helpful in reducing common vascular headaches— so called *stress* or *tension* headaches, sinus, and migraine headaches. One common cause can be caffeine, even as little as one cup of coffee can trigger headaches in sensitive individuals. A simple trial of tapering off caffeine over 10 to 14 days may help decide if this is a factor.

TABLE 5

Major Risk Factors for Heart Disease	
Cholesterol elevation	Cigarette smoking
Diabetes	Family history of premature heart disease
High blood pressure	Large amount visceral fat
Low HDL, High LDL cholesterol	Limited or no exercise
Obesity	Stress, excess and unmanaged

"Foods as causes of headaches..."

Foods as causes of headaches can sometimes be difficult to identify because sometimes the offending food may take 24 hours after being eaten to cause the headache, and it does not have to

"...fat intake ...slows stomach emptying."

happen *every time*. Be aware of some of the more common food offenders in regards to headaches: chocolate, certain cheeses (aged are the worst), nuts, monosodium glutamate (MSG), sour cream, red wine, hot dogs and other nitrite-containing meats.

Heartburn may be helped by avoiding certain foods such as citrus fruits, tomatoes, alcohol, and chocolates. Limit fat intake, since it slows stomach emptying. Don't lie down right after eating. You may also wish to try elevating the head of your bed by six inches or more with books or wooden blocks.

Body Frame Size

Although frame size has not been defined precisely, it includes body width, bone thickness, muscularity, and body proportions. There have been several methods of evaluation advocated, few of which have any standardization. One such non-standardized measurement is wrist and ankle breadth measurement.

Besides visual assessment (*eyeballing it*), another appraisal of frame size uses height:wrist circumference ratio. This ratio is found by dividing a person's height (in centimeters) by their wrist circumference (also in centi-

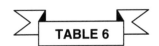

TABLE 6

How to estimate elbow breadth:

1. Place thumb and index finger on the 2 prominent bones in either side of the bent elbow.

2. Measure space between inside of the 2 fingers.

(Figures based on data from Metropolitan Life Insurance Company)

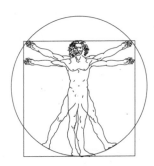

Estimation of MEDIUM Body Frame Size	
Women:	
Height (without shoes)	Elbow Breadth
4' 9" -- 4' 10"	2 1/2 -- 2 7/8"
4' 10" -- 5' 2"	2 5/8 -- 2 7/8"
5' 3" -- 5' 6"	2 3/4 -- 3"
5' 7" -- 5' 10"	2 3/4 -- 3 1/8"
5' 11" and over	2 7/8 -- 3 1/4"
Men:	
5' 1" -- 5' 2"	2 1/4 -- 2 1/2"
5' 3" -- 5' 6"	2 1/4 -- 2 1/2"
5' 7" -- 5' 10"	2 3/8 -- 2 5/8"
5' 11" -- 6' 2"	2 3/8 --2 5/8"
6' 3" and over	2 1/2 -- 2 3/4"
SMALL FRAME: Less than Medium Elbow Breadth LARGE FRAME: More than Medium Elbow Breadth	

meters). The range listed for a medium frame: men— 9.6 to 10.4; women— 10.1 to 11.0. A small frame would be for values less than those listed; large frame would be those above the stated values.

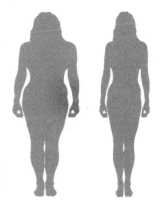

A study was performed to compare determination of small, medium, and large frame size between several methods of estimation. Visual assessment and height:wrist circumference ratio agreed with frame determination by elbow breadth measurements for less than 50% of the population. Therefore, the elbow breadth determination is considered to be a standard of choice.

A newer body frame index called **Frame Index 2** has been suggested, especially for older adults. It is determined by dividing elbow breadth (in millimeters) by body height (in centimeters) which has been multiplied by 100. Value for medium frame ages 65 to 74.9 years are: men— 40.2 to 43.4; women— 38.2 to 41.8. Small frame would consist of values less than these, and so forth.

Body Mass Index (BMI)

Using body weight as an indicator of obesity has drawbacks which have already been mentioned. A slightly better guideline (mentioned in research and epidemiological studies) which has been used in the past is the body mass index, or BMI.

The BMI is a simple measurement that has some correlation to the body's true level of fatness. It is another height- and weight-related index and can be found by dividing a person's weight (in kilograms) by their height (in meters)^2. In order to obtain kilograms, multiply weight in pounds by 0.45. To find height in meters, multiply height in inches by 0.025 (and don't forget to square the result for height — multiply it times itself to get meters squared for the denominator). If all of these calculations were too confusing, try this method: (a) multiply your weight in pounds by 700, (b) divide by your height in inches, (c) then divide by your height again. The result is your BMI.

"...weight as an indicator... has drawbacks..."

A body mass index of 25-30 kg/m^2 may be described as having low risk. Optimal weight in one study was found to correspond to the lowest of five weight categories (BMI < 22.3). An American Cancer Society study identified the lowest death rates from all causes in nonsmoking men as a BMI between 19.9-22.6; women as a BMI from 18.6-23.0. Very lean men did not show increased mortality, but rather the lowest risk of death for ischemic heart disease, cancer and stroke.

On the other hand, a BMI > 30 has been associated with a significant risk of myocardial infarction, angina pectoris and premature death. BMI of 30-35 is known to be a *moderate* risk, while one of 35-40 is considered a *high* risk. Any BMI over 40 is termed *very high* risk.

Waist-to-Hip Ratio (WHR)

Not only do we need to be concerned with the degree of body fatness for health's sake, but we must also take notice of *where* the fat is concentrated. This is because select amounts of body fat do not increase health risks—but where it is stored does (fat patterning).

The waist-to-hip ratio (WHR) allows us to characterize our fat patterning risks more precisely. It is obtained by measuring the waist, usually in the navel area, and dividing the result by the hip measurement at the largest point. (The good news is that you can perform this measurement in inches—or metric—the units cancel out).

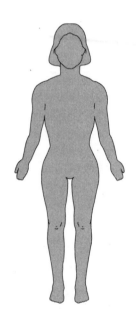

We may utilize the WHR because of its association with risk factors for ischemic heart disease, elevated serum lipids, insulin resistance, diabetes, stroke and death. In men, the risks for these problems increase dramatically when the WHR rises above 1.0 (some say 0.95) and in women when it rises above 0.80. A rule of thumb is the higher the WHR, the greater the risk.

Inherited metabolic characteristics influence the deposition of new fat in specific anatomical areas. Body fat distribution is highly correlated with gender (sex) and family genetic makeup. Males typically have a predilection to storing fat abdominally (upper body; android; central; 'apple shape'). Females tend to store fat peripherally (lower body; gynoid; femoral-gluteal; hip-thigh; 'pear shape') though there can be varying amounts and overlap in both groups.

"...WHR ...association with risk factors..."

Certain ethnic groups, such as Black Americans and Native Americans, are more prone to abdominal obesity. Black adults tend to have a more dangerous pattern of body fat patterning than white adults.

For a given state of obesity, the size of the abdominal fat compartment is affected by the genetic makeup of the individual. Upper body obesity is a much better predictor of cardiovascular disease (including myocardial infarction) and death than is general obesity. This type is highly associated with high blood pressure, serum lipid levels, glucose tolerance, diabetes, stroke, ischemic heart disease, and premature death. It may also be related to increased uterine, ovarian, and breast cancers.

Fat in the thighs and buttocks (lower body fat) has minor risk association. The fat in women's thighs was designed as a biological energy storehouse should a famine occur during pregnancy or breast-feeding.

This lower body fat may be harder to lose that upper body fat. This may be due to the fact that studies of regional fat deposits have shown that the fat cells in the hip and thigh regions in women were larger, have increased fat-producing enzyme activity, and break down fat less effectively than abdominal fat cells.

Women with high alcohol intake tend to have more abdominal fat (and therefore higher health risks due to it). In premenopausal women, alcohol affects the relationship of plasma androgens (predominantly male hormone) and upper body fat patterning.

Recumbent Sagittal Diameter

Even more closely related to risk factors is a newer technique that attempts to evaluate three compartments of the body: lean body mass, subcutaneous fat, and visceral fat. Part of the estimation involves measuring the front-to-back (sagittal) diameter of the abdomen at the level of the iliac crest (hip bone) in someone lying on their back. [Maybe they will call this the 'supine sagittal abdominal diameter', SSAD or 2SAD for short.]

So far, visceral fat (the fat *inside* the abdominal cavity and around the organs and intestines) seems to have greater relationship to risk factors for adiposity than other indicators, including the body mass index (BMI) or the waist-to-hip ratio (WHR). This has been verified with multiscan computed tomography (CT) scans. Watch for greater use of this measure in future research and evaluations.

Cancer Prevention

Cancer and dietary intake have a high correlation. About one-third of all cancer deaths may be associated with what we eat. Making appropriate dietary choices daily promotes good nutrition and good health. It may also reduce your risk of some types of cancer.

"Cancer and dietary intake have a high correlation."

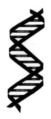

It is believed that *not smoking* is the only thing more effective than diet in reducing cancer risk. High fiber foods such as cereals and whole grain breads can be important parts of a cancer prevention diet. Other preventative measures include:

- Eating less fat and fewer animal products. Evidence is that colon and breast cancer risk may increase with a high-fat diet. In animals, fat has the highest correlation to increased cancer risk of all dietary components. Cancer-causing chemicals are stored in the fat of animals, fish and humans.
- Eating dark green leafy vegetables and yellow-orange fruits and vegetables, which contain beta-carotene and other carotenoids. These may help the body protect against cancers of the breast, bladder, mouth, larynx, and esophagus.
- Eating vegetables in the cabbage family (cruciferae or mustard), including Brussels sprouts, turnips, cauliflower, broccoli, and kale. They contain flavones, indoles, and other substances known to exhibit anti-cancer activity. Yet less than 20% of respondents in one large random survey

ate a cruciferous vegetable on the survey day. These vegetables also tend to be low cost, low-calorie, high nutrient, high fiber, and high in Vitamins A and C. Preliminary research has shown that these vitamins are associated with reduced cancer risk. In the same study mentioned, almost 75% of the study population did not include a vitamin A- or vitamin C-rich fruit or vegetable in the day's diet.

Besides dietary factors, excess weight seems to have an association with certain cancers. Obese males, regardless of smoking habits, have higher death rates from cancer of the colon, prostate, and rectum than normal weight males. Females with obesity show higher mortality from cancer of the biliary passages, gallbladder, cervix, uterus, ovaries, and breast (postmenopausal). General cancer risk is found to be much higher for obese women after menopause.

"Fat distribution also increases cancer risks."

Fat distribution also increases cancer risks. Abdominal fat distribution (central, upper body, android; 'apple shape') was predictive of breast cancer risk independently of the degree of excess weight. The prevalence of this upper body patterning in women seems to increase with age, therefore this increased risk tended to be in older women. Upper body obesity is also a risk factor in uterine (endometrial) cancer.

Are just overweight persons at higher risk from certain cancers? No, not necessarily. Lean (thin) men and women had the highest death rates from lung cancer. Lean men also had higher mortality from cancer of the bladder than men at higher weights.

Guidelines — Various Organizations

This section contains some of the guidelines advocated by the indicated organizations. These are not all encompassing but represent some of the ones relating to diet and healthy lifestyle which are summarized as follows:

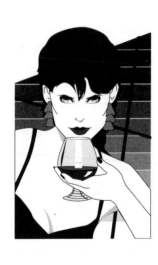

The Dietary Guidelines Advisory Committee for Americans has suggested:

(1) Eat a variety of foods
(2) Maintain desirable weight
(3) Avoid too much fat
(4) Eat foods with adequate starch and fiber
(5) Avoid too much sugar
(6) Avoid too much sodium
(7) If you drink alcoholic beverages, do so in moderation

The National Institutes of Health consensus panel recommends:

• blood cholesterol level < 180 mg/dL if less than 30 years old
• blood cholesterol level < 200 mg/dL if older than 30

The American Heart Association recommends:

- 4 or more servings of vegetables and fruits (or juices)
- 4 or more servings of bread, cereal, and starchy foods
- 2 or more servings of lowfat milk, cheese and dairy products
- 5-7 oz of lean meat, fish, or poultry
- no more than 5-8 teaspoons of fats and oils
- eat more egg whites and limit whole eggs or egg yolks to no more than two per week
- eat other lowfat, low-cholesterol foods
- restrict total dietary fat to 30% of intake with polyunsaturated and saturated fat no more than 10% of daily totals each
- 1 gram sodium (1000 mg) per 1000 calorie daily intake, not to exceed 3 grams daily (if normal blood pressure)
- limit cholesterol intake to 100 mg per 1000 calorie intake, not to exceed 300 mg per day
- for those consuming alcohol, drink no more than 1 and 1/2 oz of pure alcohol daily (3 oz of 100-proof whiskey, two 12 oz beers, or two 4 oz glasses of wine)

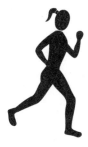

The **Council on Fitness** recommends a minimum of 20 minutes of sustained activity at least three times a week in order to obtain the cardiovascular and respiratory benefits of aerobic activity. This should be in addition to a five minute warm-up and five minute cool-down.

The **American College of Sports Medicine** recommends exercising 35-60 minutes three to five times per week for cardiovascular conditioning. During the workout, you should be using large muscle groups in a continuous, rhythmic fashion.

Health Factors

Health is such a broad topic that it could not be covered adequately in one book, much less in this short section. In fact, many sections of this book touch on health topics and healthy eating and could be considered subsets of this category. Since even something as simple as a ten pound weight loss in certain hypertensives might significantly reduce their blood pressure, we will focus on weight reduction and maintenance tips as the primary thrust of this section.

There can be many rewards that come from weight loss and maintenance of that loss. Your own list will probably surpass these but perhaps they will get you thinking.

"...excess weight carries greater risk..."

Many of the benefits may be *Hidden*. Some of the chronic disease states for which excess weight carries greater risk may be milder or nonexistent with weight reduction. Feeling better, having more energy, increased stamina, and the like are usually less tangible to others than smaller clothes sizes.

An improved *Attitude* may be another benefit. And why shouldn't it be better when our excess bulges shrink and our clothes fit better? If you use the proper frame of mind, you will succeed.

Our *Personal fitness* should also be enhanced. The increased activities of daily living should improve muscle tone, increase circulation, and strengthen heart performance.

Pleasure in doing something you enjoy. This comes from making healthy changes gradually and utilizing substitutions instead of sacrifices. You can be pleased at your accomplishments and be proud of the way you have finally taken charge of your lifestyle and behavior.

If you feel *Younger*, then you are experiencing another potential benefit of adopting a healthy lifestyle, complemented by appropriate exercise and weight management.

We can build the acronym *HAPPY* from the first letters of these potential weight management rewards. Don't we all want to be *HAPPY*? Good health will certainly help us work towards that goal.

How do we keep this *HAPPY feeling*? A partial answer would be to stay successful in our weight reduction and maintenance. And how do we do that, considering the national statistics regarding maintenance of weight lost are dismal (<5-10% successful over 1-5 years)? Our best research to date identifies at least five areas to help improve your chances of successful weight control. They are as follows:

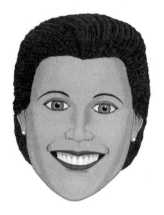

"...knowledge seems to be a key for intelligent people."

1) Behavior modification— helps identify and change unhealthy habits, attitudes, eating and lifestyle patterns.

2) Nutrition education— knowledge seems to be a key for intelligent people. We need to understand the importance and reasoning behind the new basic food groups, portion control, calories, fat content, and what constitutes sensible weight management goals and guidelines.

3) Self-Monitoring— recording food intake (food diary), weight, measurements, exercise type and frequency helps focus attention on weight loss and control and re-enforces positive behavioral changes.

4) Exercise— increases muscle tone and sense of well-being, burns calories, provides diversion to eating, allows sense of accomplishment, and builds self-esteem.

5) Support Network— continued periodic contact with family, friends, community support group and/or health care professionals has a high

correlation with successful weight maintenance. Being accountable to someone else gives you motivation and encourages successful weight loss and maintenance.

Special Concerns

When questioned about their most important reasons for desiring weight loss, many people cited concerns about their future and concerns about their current *appearance* (#1 reason), *fitness* (#2), and *health* (farther down the list). Women saw appearance as more important than fitness, while men rated fitness over appearance. Wanting to lose weight gained after stopping smoking or pregnancy were other reasons cited.

"...there are ...risks associated with weight reduction..."

While these are all valid reasons for wanting to reduce weight, an informed person needs to be aware that there are also certain risks associated with weight reduction, *just as there may be certain benefits*. Weight cycling (gain-lose cycle) has been shown to increase health risks and may be related to development of chronic disease. Therefore, weight reduction is not without potential hazard or risk (especially in programs not utilizing sensible methods). Even using *phenylpropanolamine* (PPA), a common ingredient in many over-the-counter dieting aids and cold remedies, has been associated with fatal strokes, dangerously high blood pressure, cardiac irregularities, heart muscle and kidney damage, psychosis, headaches, seizures, hallucinations, nervousness and insomnia.

It may be a *Catch 22* situation whereby you feel trapped and frustrated either way. This emphasizes the importance of discussion of your weight management program with a trained health care professional, preferably your physician.

The following risks are just some of the ones known to be attributed to weight loss and do not constitute a listing of every risk possible:

CAUTION
WATCH YOUR STEP

- abdominal pain
- aching muscles
- amenorrhea and decreased libido
- anemia
- both slowed and increased heart rate
- cardiac disorders
- changes in liver function
- cold intolerance

- death
- diarrhea, constipation
- dry skin
- edema (fluid in tissues)
- elevated cholesterol
- elevated uric acid levels
- fainting, weakness and fatigue
- gallstones
- gouty arthritis

- hair loss and thinning hair (usually temporary)
- headache
- hypotension (low blood pressure)
- loss of lean tissue
- muscle cramps
- nausea

In addition to the potential side effects already mentioned, **rapid** weight loss can also cause:

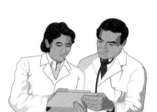

"...rapid weight loss can also cause... dehydration"

- abnormal increase in fibrous connective tissue in vital organs due to repeated attempts at weight loss using starvation methods
- anemia, characterized by fatigue, weakness, paleness, reduced resistance to infection, lowered exercise ability and diminished attention span
- dehydration
- dizziness when standing or turning quickly
- electrolyte imbalance, such as low body potassium or sodium, which may lead to heart irregularities
- emotional stress, perplexity, anxiousness or depression
- increased blood uric acid levels, which can cause or exacerbate gout or uric acid kidney stones
- overeating— binge frequency may be higher
- poor long-term weight maintenance, especially if original behavior and lifestyle not permanently modified
- temporary skin rash
- unusual pressure in the nerves of the leg which can lead to numbness or loss of muscle strength

There has been concern regarding rapid weight loss and the development of gallstones due to supersaturation of biliary cholesterol and gallbladder stasis. Cause and effect are still being investigated but one group of researchers has made a suggestion to help lower such potential risk. They feel that a diet that has sufficient protein (i.e., 14 grams) and fat (i.e., 10 grams) at *one meal* will ensure gallbladder contraction. They also recommend limiting weight reduction to 2% or less of body weight per week.

Some obesity specialists say that fast weight loss is dangerous in and of itself. They feel that if weight is lost too rapidly, the body draws too much from its own lean mass. Others think adequate protein intake during weight reduction can help prevent or reduce this problem. Lean loss is important to be aware of because we know loss of lean tissue can disturb heart function and damage other organs.

"...thin folks tend to lose more lean mass..."

It has been found that weight loss in lean individuals leads to a greater proportion of lean body mass loss than in severely overweight persons (thin folks tend to lose more lean mass than obese weight reducers). The actual amount of lean mass lost during weight reduction depends on at least four factors: (1) dietary intake percentages and quality of proteins and carbohydrates, (2) duration of weight reducing phase, (3) initial body fat content, and (4) the calorie deficit.

During the early 1970's, there were at least 58 documented deaths of persons on liquid protein diets, and six deaths in the early 1980's from the

Cambridge diet. The Michigan Task Force lists sudden and potentially fatal heart irregularities (cardiac arrhythmias) as risks of diets utilizing less than 800 calories.

It should be mentioned that several epidemiological studies have raised the association of weight loss with increased mortality. However, it must also be stated that in several of them, the *reason* weight was lost is unknown. For example, it would make a *big difference* if the subjects lost weight due to a chronic illness, had cancer or acquired immunodeficiency syndrome, or had lost weight due to smoking.

"Quitting smoking doesn't have to be a weight disaster."

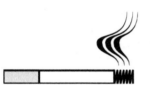

Of equal importance to health is the consideration of smoking, especially when used as a form of weight control or if continued because of a fear of weight gain. Smoking (nicotine) is probably the most commonly used—and dangerous—weight control drug of all. In one study, twenty percent of overweight women smokers had started smoking as a form of weight control because of nicotine increasing metabolism. The National Institutes of Health suggests that people who smoke for weight control should be aware that (1) their fat distribution is likely to be of the more dangerous android (upper body) kind, and (2) if they quit smoking they may gain some weight, but the fat patterning is likely to improve (thereby decreasing other medical risks).

When weight is gained after smoking cessation, it is usually through intake of extra food and the body being more efficient, thereby requiring fewer calories for weight gain. Sensible, lowfat eating and increased activity can help offset this increased weight tendency. (*It is a lot healthier to be a little overweight than to be a smoker.*)

Quitting smoking doesn't have to be a weight disaster. One study showed that men and women ex-smokers generally gained up to the average weight of persons who had never smoked. The average gain for men was six pounds and for women was eight pounds.

Diabetes

What is diabetes and why is it listed in a weight management manual? I'll answer the second half of the question first. There seems to be a high correlation between obesity and adult onset non-insulin dependent diabetes mellitus. Many patients (70%) with this disorder are overweight at the time of diagnosis. It is theorized that if people maintained *normal* weight, many potential diabetics might delay the onset of this disease or avoid it altogether. Also, weight control can often reduce the severity of diabetes.

"Diabetes affects some 12 million Americans..."

Diabetes affects some 12 million Americans, almost half of whom don't even realize they have it. It is a disorder whereby the body has trouble handling *carbohydrates* (starches and sugars). After they are eaten and digested, they are changed into a simple sugar—glucose.

"Nutrition is important in controlling diabetes..."

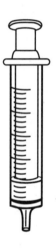

In order to utilize the energy of glucose, the body needs a hormone produced in the pancreas called *insulin*. Insulin is released into the bloodstream after a meal to help muscle, liver, and other cells use and store the glucose. When those cells are full, insulin forces glucose into the fat cells in the form of a fat called triglyceride. However, diabetics don't produce enough insulin or else the individual's cells become less sensitive to its effects. Whichever the case (or a combination of both), not all of the glucose is used. The excess builds up in the blood and causes *elevated blood sugar* (hyperglycemia) and some slips past the filters of the kidney to cause sugar (glucose) in the urine.

Some of these problems can present with symptoms of excess hunger and thirst, frequent urination, and tiredness. Diabetes can cause damage to many of the body's organ systems, including the blood vessels in the heart, nerve damage, kidney damage, hypertension, and loss of vision. Some diabetics have elevated triglycerides (building blocks for cholesterol) and lowered levels of the *good* HDL cholesterol. Severe medical complications may ultimately develop, including premature death. The death rate for those who develop diabetes after age 40, is two to three times higher than the general population. Cardiovascular disease is a high contributor to this increased risk of mortality.

Nutrition is important in controlling diabetes once it has been acquired. Controlling diabetes through proper nutrition may prevent some diseases associated with this ailment and may slow the progression of kidney, nerve, and eye damage. The American Dietetic Association recommends that diabetics follow a diet containing 20 percent protein, 50 to 60 percent carbohydrate, and less than 30 percent fat. High-fiber diets are usually suggested to help them lower *bad* LDL and total cholesterol.

One suspected link between diabetes and excess weight is that excess weight gain in adulthood may be more likely to result in upper body adiposity (fat distribution) and enlarged fat cells. In turn, this might lead to insulin resistance (lower cell sensitivity) and hyperinsulinemia (elevated insulin levels).

Several other things can affect the risk of acquiring diabetes. The rate of diabetes is 50 percent higher among black females than in whites. Also, people who use exercise as their only means of controlling weight were able to reduce their risk of developing diabetes compared to staying overweight.

DIETS

General Info & Risks

Before we delve into a discussion of *diets*, let's look at some of the statistics regarding dieting, weight loss, and the industry in general.

"Diets...are not just about eating."

- Dieting and health spas are a multi-billion dollar industry in the United States.
- There are almost 30,000 methods of weight loss, but less than 6% are considered safe or effective.
- At any given time, almost 10 million Americans are in some type of weight program.
- Almost 50% of women and 25% of men are trying to lose weight at any given time (many of which are not overweight).
- Each year, two-thirds of the population report going on at least one or more diets.
- The average dieter goes on about 2 diets a year. Women dieters average 3 per year.
- Studies examining dieting among teenagers show from 44-62% of girls and 15-28% of boys (depending upon the survey) have dieted in the past year—many using potentially harmful methods.
- About 90% of weight-reducers are back to their original weights within one year; almost 95% by five years.

"Nutritionally... best diet is... a variety of foods..."

Diets and dieting are not just about *eating*. They involve an entire way of life. Since we usually associate dieting with eating (or lack of), we need new terminology and a fresh perspective. I will continue to mention the **D**-*word* (diet), but only to show its negativity, inadequacy, and dangers. In addition to physical damage, the dangers of dieting include emotional and psychological harm, eating disorders, financial cost, and reduced lifestyle potential. It really should be eliminated from our vocabulary.

As we leave diets behind, think instead of conscious, deliberate *food choices.*

- Think *substitution* instead of *sacrifice*.
- Think *modification* instead of *masochism*.
- Think *alternatives* instead of *anorexia*.
- Think *resourceful* instead of *restrictions*.
- Think *selections* instead of *starvation*.
- Think *fun* instead of *forbidden*.
- Think *can* instead of *cannot*.

Avoid all fad and crash diets. They are just that— a diet. Most fad diets are nutritionally inadequate, scientifically unsound, expensive, and potentially dangerous. They do nothing to change defective eating habits. After they are over, the old habits and food attitudes will return you to the old (high-fat) way of eating and probably the old weight as well. Instead, change the normal foods you eat to lower-fat through gradual substitution and modification. Nutritionally, the best diet is to eat a variety of foods drawn from the basic food groups (see Pyramid Guide page 126).

Unfortunately, many obese persons think that restrictive dieting is the road to successful weight control. However, it can lead to loss of control, overeating, and cycles of repeat dieting with weight fluctuation. This is verified when almost 40 percent of all obese patients presenting for treatment suffer from binge eating disorder, characterized by frequent and uncontrollable binge eating.

Weight management is not an issue of restrictions and weight reduction but of *lifestyle* and *behavioral changes*. An effective weight management program (such as this one) will incorporate: (1) sensible eating (vs. dieting), (2) increased activity, (3) behavior changes targeted to control over-eating or bingeing, (4) motivation, and (5) positive thinking.

Anecdotal evidence shows that persons successful in losing and maintaining weight make *gradual shifts* in their eating style towards lower fat foods, without feelings of deprivation and sacrifice. You may need to eat regular meals with snacks for awhile to get out of the bingeing cycle. Do what it takes to abandon the *diet* mentality.

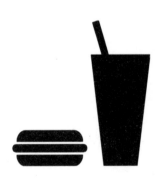

Dietary changes are the most commonly used weight loss strategies. Methods run the gambit from restricting calories to changing percentage intake from fats, proteins, and carbohydrates. The size of the calorie reduction and composition of the diet can change the mix of metabolic fuels that are burned for energy, the type of tissue lost, body water balance, and weight lost.

"Low carbohydrate diets don't work..."

Just changing the percentage intake of nutrients has an effect on weight loss. However, the effects seem small in comparison with the direct effect of caloric restriction. The same can be said about exercise too. Reducing calories consumed enhances weight reduction beyond that of exercise alone.

Low carbohydrate diets don't work for several reasons. Glycogen, the storage form of carbohydrate requires 4 grams of water for every 1 gram stored. Weight loss diets utilizing low carbohydrates work by depleting your glycogen stores. Most of the weight lost is the water used to store the glycogen, not the fat stores hoped for. The loss may be quick, but it is temporary.

Successful maintainers typically achieve a weight that is about halfway between their starting weight and the *ideal* weight from charts. Some take weight reduction breaks after losing some weight. This helps build confidence and allows them to work on behavior at one level before proceeding to the next level of modification.

One suggestion that may help with weight management is to give away or alter your clothes as soon as they become too large. If you don't, this is giving yourself *permission* to regain the lost weight. Eating a meal in clothes that are a little snug around the waist is one of the best reminders for sensible eating that you can have.

"...moderation seems to be the key."

There are several other things to consider. Female athletes and women who *diet severely* can disrupt their reproductive ability because of very low body fat. This tends to affect their hormone status. On the other hand, a very high percentage of body fat can also cause infertility.

Much evidence suggests that being slightly under so-called *ideal weight* improves mortality rates. However, many experts believe it is unhealthy to be too thin. Since disagreement abounds, moderation seems to be the key.

Starvation

Total starvation results in very large losses of *lean body tissue* and is not recommended as an obesity therapy. Lean body mass loss can approach as much as 50-60% of the weight lost, especially in leaner individuals. With a total fast, the proportion of weight lost during the second week onward is about one-half fat and one-half lean body mass (non-fat).

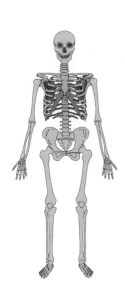

Both fasting and very-low-calorie diets (VLCDs) are drastic weight loss measures that have extreme metabolic effects. They cause water, sodium, and potassium losses. Certain nutrients have to be supplemented in VLCDs to increase their safety.

Starvation is self-defeating because the large lean body mass loss usually causes a reduction in basal (resting) metabolic rate. This leads to less calories being burned overall and less weight loss.

> **FICTION:** Fasting is a great way to lose weight, especially when you have a timetable to meet.
> **FACT:** Fasting can have detrimental effects on liver and kidney function, cause accelerated loss of muscle and non-fat tissue, and when carried to extreme, can change the chemical balance in the blood (electrolytes, blood sugar, etc.). Those who lose weight by fasting are more apt to regain it. A better method is to learn how to modify eating habits, change inappropriate behavior, and adopt a healthier lifestyle.

NUTRITION

Calories

The calorie (actually the kilocalorie) is the amount of heat required to raise the temperature of one liter of water (approximately 1 quart) by 1 degree Celsius. The caloric value of any food is a measure of the energy available to the body—just like the inch is a measure of length. Calories also measure energy *used* by the body, or *burned* (as in activity).

Calories in food are derived from three nutrients: proteins, carbohydrates, and fats. Vitamins, minerals, and water provide no calories but are essential to the body's production of energy. The following are calories per gram in selected items:

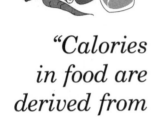

- **Proteins**: 4 calories per gram
- **Carbohydrates**: 4 calories per gram
- **Fats**: 9 calories per gram
- **Alcohol**: 7 calories per gram
- **Vitamins** & **Minerals**: nil calories
- **Water**: nil calories

"Calories in food are derived from 3 nutrients..."

Note that fats have over *twice* the energy value of protein and carbohydrate. Thus, the higher the fat (or oil) content of food, the higher the calories. Excess calories (whether from fats, carbohydrates or protein) are stored as body fat. However, there is evidence that the body stores dietary *fats* easier and quicker into our own fat cells than proteins and carbohydrates.

Some sample calculations of food calorie values are as follows:

Chicken McNuggets has 288 calories derived from:

20 grams protein (x4cal/gm)	= 80 calories
17.24 gm carbohydrate (x4cal/gm)	= 69 calories
15.44 gm fat (x9cal/gm)	= 139 calories
Total Calories (6 nuggets)	= 288 calories

Red Lobster dry-broiled Mackerel has 192 calories derived from:

20 grams protein (x4cal/gm)	= 80 calories
1 gm carbohydrate (x4cal/gm)	= 4 calories
12 gm fat (x9cal/gm)	= 108 calories
Total Calories (5 oz.)	= 192 calories

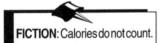

FICTION: Calories do not count.

FACT: They do count. Your present weight is partially the difference between calories taken in vs. calories used up.

Our bodies use calories for every activity, whether at work, play, or sleeping. Many observers feel that the heavier you are, the more energy you use— though this has been disputed by some studies. Food is the *fuel* we use to feed our body's energy demands and should be monitored to allow balancing our energy requirements.

To maintain weight, food calories taken in should balance calories expended by the body. To lose weight, more calories should be used than taken in. Often quoted is the requirement of ***3,500 calories*** needed per pound of fat. If loss of a pound of fat a week is desired, you need a deficit of about 500 calories per day—

either through eating this much less or by increasing activity by this amount or a combination of the two.

Be cautious about reducing calories too much as the body seems to become more energy-efficient with continued calorie restriction. Studies have indicated that reducing daily caloric intake below 800 kcal/day does not increase the amount of fat lost. In fact, there seems to be little benefit to severely restricting calorie intake as subjects on either a 420, 660, or 800 kcal daily diet showed only marginal differences in their weight losses. Hunger breakthrough seems to one major drawback.

Low-calorie diets are usually used in mildly overweight patients (body mass index 25-30). They tend to provide from 800 to 1300 calories per day.

Very-low-calorie diets (VLCDs) are defined by an intake equal to or below 800 calories per day. Because of potential risks involved with these diets, many feel they should be limited to patients a minimum of 50 pounds overweight (more than 130% of ideal body weight). They should provide a minimum of 70 grams of protein a day (or 1.2-1.5 grams protein/kilogram ideal body weight) and adjusted to restrict lean body mass loss to 15% or less of weight being lost.

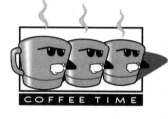

When it comes to calories, it is sometimes the things we consider insignificant that trip us up. Take for example a morning ritual of two cups of coffee, each with two lumps of sugar and two tablespoons of creamer. This can be almost 300 calories. In contrast, the same two cups with artificial sweetener and skim milk provide only about one-tenth the amount of calories. Be alert for high caloric foods and condiments and learn to substitute and avoid these sneaky calories.

"Nothing tastes as good as thin feels!"

Have you ever been tempted by the cocktail peanuts sitting on the coffee table or at the bar in a restaurant? They are some of the worst nuts (calories & fats) for weight managers as one ounce has 166 calories. Consume a bowlful and you can sock away 1,000 calories without thinking, even before you have had dinner.

When these or other temptations arise, remember: *Nothing tastes as good as thin feels!* That should help get you back to meeting your healthful goals—or at least keep you from deviating too far.

FOOD GROUPS

Like any successful project, weight loss and management works better when you have a plan. Part of the planning for healthful eating should include knowledge and use of food groups. In general, consumption of over half your intake from complex carbohydrates, 15-20% from proteins, and no more than 30% of intake from fats (preferably lower) will keep you within suggested guidelines. You may wish to utilize a food diary to help you calculate and analyze caloric intake to assure it contains the appropriate groups and has adequate calories.

There has been a lot of concern recently about the old *basic four food groups*. It has been felt that the old guidelines emphasized too much high-fat meat and dairy products at the expense of our long-term health. The new four groups listed below come from the *Physicians Committee for Responsible Medicine*. They reflect the massive research telling us that the more we consume meat and dairy products, the more we suffer from illness and poor health.

The new four food groups consist of grains, legumes, fruits, and vegetables. These recommendations should be used in conjunction with the *Eating Right Pyramid* found on pages 126-127.

The Physicians Committee groups and serving recommendations are as follows:

"Choose whole fruit over fruit juices..."

1. **Whole grains (5 or more servings a day);** Serving size: 1/2 cup hot cereal; 1 oz. dry cereal; 1 slice of bread
2. **Legumes (2 to 3 servings a day);** Serving size: 1/2 cup cooked beans; 4 oz. tofu or tempeh; 8 oz. soy milk
3. **Vegetables (3 or more servings a day);** Serving size: 1 cup raw; 1/2 cup cooked; and
4. **Fruits (3 or more servings a day).** Serving size: 1 medium piece of fruit; 1/2 cup cooked fruit; 1/2 cup fruit juice

The first group, *whole grains*, includes bread, rice, pasta, hot or cold cereal, corn, millet, barley, bulgur, buckwheat and tortillas. It is recommended to build each meal around a hearty grain dish. Grains are rich in fiber and other complex carbohydrates, as well as protein, B-vitamins and zinc.

Legumes, the next grouping, is another name for beans, peas, and lentils, which are all good sources of fiber, protein, iron, calcium, zinc and B-vitamins. This group also includes chickpeas, baked and refried beans, soy milk, tofu, tempeh, and texturized vegetable protein.

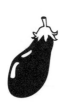

Vegetables are the third major group. They are packed with nutrients and provide vitamin C, beta-carotene, riboflavin and other vitamins, iron, calcium and fiber. Dark green, leafy vegetables such as broccoli, collards, kale, mustard and turnip greens, chicory or bok choy are especially good sources of these important nutrients. Dark yellow and orange vegetables such as carrots, winter squash, sweet potatoes and pumpkin provide extra beta-carotene. Include generous portions of a variety of vegetables in your diet.

The last major grouping by the Physicians Committee are *fruits*. Fruits are rich in fiber, vitamin C and beta-carotene. Be sure to include at least one serving each day of fruits that are high in vitamin C—citrus fruits, melons and strawberries are all good choices. Choose whole fruit over fruit juices, which don't contain as much healthy fiber.

Protein

1 gram = 4 calories

Protein includes any one of a group of complex organic nitrogen-containing compounds. Simply stated, protein provides us with amino acids and nitrogen, necessary ingredients for life. These are used to build and repair body tissues, including muscle. Proteins are also the building blocks of our body's hormones, enzymes, antibodies, and organs.

"Plant proteins are not inferior..."

There are 22 biologically important amino acids, 8 of which are not synthesized by humans in life-sustaining quantities and must be supplied through dietary intake—but only small amounts of animal foods (preferably lowfat) need be eaten, if at all. (Infants do require some form of milk in their diet to obtain sufficient protein and calories). It is easy to obtain adequate protein in our dietary intake, even on a vegetarian diet. Plant proteins are not inferior to animal proteins.

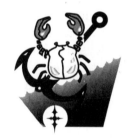

When not trying to lose weight, we may need less daily protein than was once thought important. The World Health Organization, the Food and Nutrition Board of the National Academy of Sciences, and the National Research Council say that we only need a maximum of 8% of our total daily calories from protein (and this includes a *safety factor* of an extra 30%). You may actually only need about 6% of total calories as protein—it is very difficult to get below 9% with *ordinary* dietary intake.

Concern about adequate protein intake is probably not warranted with a healthy and varied diet. Even an infant (who grows at an extremely fast rate) is best served nutritionally with mother's breast milk—which only provides 5% of its calories as protein. The average American consumes 90-120 grams of protein per day, while the ideal protein intake for humans has been stated to be about 20-40 grams per day.

"...weight loss should be unhurried..."

During times we are trying to lose weight we may slip into negative protein (and nitrogen) balance, which can cause some loss of lean body mass. Although some lean body mass is almost always lost when fat tissue is lost, assuring that protein intake is sufficient can minimize these losses.

Protein is an emergency fuel for the body in the absence of adequate carbohydrates and fats. For this reason, weight loss should be unhurried so as to preserve protein levels in muscle, the heart, and other body organs. Some sources use a rule of thumb for protein intake of at least 1.5 gram per kilogram ideal body weight per day (nearly 20% of total calories on a conventional 800 calorie diet) to help maintain lean body mass and spare body nitrogen. Other guides list a protein level of 0.8-1.0 gm/kg ideal body weight. However, the best advice when on restricted calorie intake is to consult your supervising physician for their recommendations.

Although muscles are built of protein, protein itself is not a special fuel for working muscle cells—carbohydrates and fatty acids are. Protein combustion is no higher during heavy exercise than under resting conditions. In fact, a diet high in protein (and fat) with little carbohydrate, can significantly reduce the performance of an athlete involved in endurance sports. Don't forget that excess protein intake will not build bigger muscles. It is converted in our bodies and stored as fat.

There are many potential sources of protein, some of which we will discuss in the following paragraphs. There may be some overlap with the section on *Fats* as many animal sources of protein also contain fats and can be discussed under either group.

FISH

Fish can be a very good choice for healthy eating as it is a great source of protein. It has about as much protein as red meat, but a lot less fat. For example, a six ounce T-bone steak has about 555 calories and 42 grams of fat (378 calories from fat). Six ounces of dry-broiled flounder has about 115 calories and less than one gram of fat (about 7 or 8 fat calories). Fish fat is rich in vitamins A and D (needed for healthy bones, teeth, skin, and eyes). The meaty portions of fish supply the B vitamins.

Seafood can be a great supplement to soups, salads, pasta dishes, and other main entrees. Fish oils tend to be polyunsaturated and may help lower blood triglyceride and cholesterol levels. Another potential benefit is that many kinds of fish contain a polyunsaturated fat called eicosapentaneoic acid (EPA), which acts as a blood thinner and can reduce the potential for blood clots that often lead to heart attacks. However, fish oils (omega-3 fatty acids) may also raise the rate of hemorrhagic strokes and the incidence of impotence. Some studies have also shown fish oils to interfere with the function of the human immune system's natural killer cells. Therefore, it might be wise to refrain from going overboard with taking megadoses of fish oil in those gelatin capsules you find at the health food store.

TABLE 7

Kind of Fish	Fat Grams per 4 oz. serving
Cod, dolphin, flounder, haddock, lobster, scallops and sole	< 1
Grouper, pike, pollock	1.0 - 1.3
Monkfish, ocean perch, rockfish, shrimp, snapper	1.5 - 2.0
Orange roughy	8.0
Butterfish, Pacific mackerel	8.9
Sockeye salmon	9.7
Atlantic herring	10.3
Chinook salmon	11.9
Atlantic mackerel, Pacific herring	15.7
Sablefish	17.3

"Fish oils tend to be polyunsaturated..."

TRUE or FALSE: Tuna canned in oil has over *ten times* the fat content of tuna packed in water.
(True)
Water-packed tuna is about 3% fat compared to 36% fat in oil-packed.)

Choose fresh or frozen fillets, or canned fish packed in water. Avoid fried fish, frozen fish in batter, or canned fish in oil. Fish sticks can often be hidden sources of fat. You may wish to limit shrimp and squid somewhat due to higher cholesterol (though some controversy exists). Crayfish and shrimp have about double the cholesterol as meat but much less fat. The fat they do have is mostly unsaturated and contains heart-healthy omega-3 fatty acids.

There are some valid concerns regarding whether our commercial fish supply is really safe, considering all the pollution that abounds worldwide. It is difficult to find fish from unpolluted waters. The Center for Science in the Public Interest suggests that cod, haddock, pollock, and salmon are likely to be the safer fish choices.

CHICKEN

Chicken can be a very good eating selection on a lowfat diet. It is very low in saturated fat compared to other meats, but is still high in cholesterol. If you only eat the white meat of the chicken, without the skin, and cook it with non-fat cooking methods such as baking, dry grilling, roasting, broiling, or steaming you can greatly reduce the amount of fat in your meal. White meat chicken has less fats and calories than the dark meat. However, its lowfat benefits can easily be reversed if it is prepared improperly.

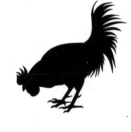

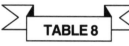

TABLE 8

"Chicken can be a very good eating selection..."

Non-Fried Chicken	
White or Dark	*Fat Grams per 4 oz. Serving*
Drumstick roasted w/o skin	6.4
Thigh roasted w/o skin	12.4
Breast roasted w/o skin	4.1
Breast roasted w/ skin	8.8
Fried Chicken	
How Prepared	*Fat Grams per 4 oz. Serving*
Breast fried with skin, flour-coated	10.1
Breast fried with skin, batter dipped	20.7
Breast prepared at fast food restaurant	27.4

By removing the skin, you remove a lot of chicken's excess fats. For example, by removing the skin from a chicken breast, you can cut its fat content by more than half. Some sources state that it may not matter [fat-wise] whether your remove the skin before or after cooking. Either way, vertical baking or roasting of poultry keeps fat content down.

Skin also becomes an important consideration in ground chicken. One pound of commercially ground chicken (typically includes the skin as *filler*) has about 60 fat grams per pound. If you purchase skinless white meat chicken and have it ground to order it is only about 15 fat grams per pound (about 1/4 as much as commercial ground and packaged).

Compared to ground beef at 96 fat grams per pound, chicken is a good choice. Chicken breast meat is the lowest in fat and perhaps your best chicken choice. One six ounce roasted chicken breast without the skin is about 6 fat grams versus six ounces of ground beef at 36 fat grams.

Good judgment in the manner of preparation is critical to lowfat eating. One-half of a chicken breast without skin is only 3 fat grams. If you roast it with skin, the same piece more than doubles its fat, to about 7.6 fat grams. Fry it with a batter coating and you more than double it again, to over 17 fat grams. Using dark meat in this last example (frying with batter) increases your count to 20-25 fat grams.

TURKEY

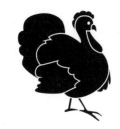

Another lowfat poultry selection is turkey. It is actually lower in fat than chicken and definitely lower fat (especially saturated fat) than hamburger or beef. Therefore, it makes a great lowfat substitute for beef in many food items and main dishes. Turkey cutlets can be used instead of veal cutlets. It can be ground and used to replace hamburger meat in tacos, lasagna, chili, meat loaf, spaghetti sauce, casseroles or for a pizza topping.

As an informed consumer and a wise, heart-healthy eater, knowing some of the pitfalls of purchasing and selecting turkey becomes important. You may be able to find cello-wrapped, ground in-store turkey, sometimes at a price less than a commercial brand of ground turkey. Beware though because the in-store brand probably has the highest fat content of any ground turkey, consisting of fat, skin, dark meat, and white meat. In some cases, it may even be higher in fat than the lean ground beef a few partitions over.

The benefit of selecting a commercial brand of ground turkey over the cello-wrapped version is that it typically contains a nutrition label listing ingredients and fat content. Commercial compa-

TABLE 9

"...turkey ...lower in fat than chicken..."

Turkey	
How Prepared	**Fat Grams per 4 oz. Serving**
Ground white meat without skin	1.3
White meat (breast) without skin	1.3
White meat without skin	3.6
Butterball white meat without skin	4.6
Butterball dark meat without skin	11.4
Dark meat without skin	8
Ground turkey (90% lean)	8

nies also use a mixture of dark and white meat in their ground turkey packages, and this can lead to fairly high fat content too. For example, one pound of Armour Turkey Select packaged ground turkey contains 32 fat grams.

Is this the best we can do? Not by a long shot. The best selection is to select packages of white meat turkey breasts, have the butcher remove the skin, and grind it for you while you wait. Most butchers will be pleased to do this for you and the little extra time spent waiting for this service saves you a tremendous amount of calories and fat. One pound of fresh ground white turkey breasts, without the skin, is only about 5.3 fat grams. This is a difference of 26.7 fat grams per pound over the commercial brands (and a lot more over the in-store cello packages).

A few extra tips regarding turkey are in order. If you wish to lower calories and fat intake, select white meat over dark meat. Also, try to use plain turkeys rather than the Butterball or similar brands (which tend to have higher fat content). Since turkey has little fat compared to the amount of protein present, it tends to cook quicker than you might expect. Follow appropriate cooking directions and avoid overcooking, as this will make it tough.

BEEF

Beef and red meats should be very low on our list of protein selections, mainly because of the associated fats, many of which are saturated and considered unhealthy. Generally, the higher the grade of beef, the more fat it contains. Commercial grades of meat are generally rated as follows:
- **Prime** — contains the most fats   • **Select/Good** — least fat of meat grades
- **Choice** — less fat than prime

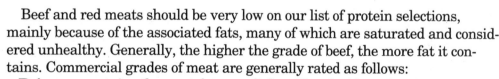

TABLE 10

Beef	
Type of Beef	**Fat Grams per 4 oz. Serving**
Golden Trim ground beef	6.6
Eye of round (roasted)	16.2
Sirloin steak (broiled)	20.6
Ribeye steak (broiled)	23.5
Porterhouse steak (broiled)	24.2
Ground beef (cooked)	24.6
T-Bone steak (broiled)	28.1
Beef Brisket (braised)	37

"...the higher the grade of beef, the more fat..."

Buy lean grades of meat and trim off visible fat before cooking. Top round, eye of round, London broil, and sirloin tip are among the leanest cuts. Broiling or roasting on an elevated drip pan can keep fats from being reabsorbed and can help reduce the fat intake. However, brisket and high grades of meat have a moderate amount of fat marbled throughout the meat that cannot be removed by cooking, so make intelligent lowfat choices whenever you eat red meat. Be aware of the cut of meat, the portion size, and how it is cooked. A wise selection could be 100% lean, choice grade flank steak, eight ounces of which is 13 fat grams. A similar eight ounce lean cut of round steak has 14 fat grams. By eating only four ounces, you can even cut this amount of fat in half. Having your butcher tenderize it for you or marinating it for several hours or overnight can certainly enhance the selection.

"...look for new lowfat products..."

Other healthy meat tips include combining meat with other foods in mixed dishes such as pasta, soup, or vegetable stew to reduce the quantity of meat consumed. Eat organ meat, such as liver, kidney, and brain, only occasionally. Also, cut down on lamb, duck, and veal as they are all quite high in saturated fat (sometimes more than beef). Other high-fat meat products to reduce include sausage, frankfurters, bacon, and salami. Choose lean luncheon meats (90% fat-free) over high fat cold cuts— but make sure the *lowfat* designation is *percent fat of total calories*, not percent of total product weight (this is a frequently used marketing trick).

Continue to look for *new* lowfat products appearing on the consumer market from time to time, such as the new Golden Trim ground beef which supposedly has 26.4 fat grams per pound (or about 1.6 fat grams per ounce). Healthy Choice ground beef is supposed to be only about 1 fat gram per ounce. Since products and brands may come and go, you need to be alert.

If you would like to remove almost half the fat from ground beef in chili, spaghetti sauce, or other recipes, try the following tip. Brown the meat in a skillet and then place it on paper towels and blot. Next, place it in a colander or strainer and rinse it with hot (not boiling) water. Finally, drain it completely and use as your recipe directs. Another way to reduce the fat would be to microwave it on a paper towel.

PORK

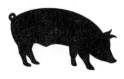

Pork is generally considered a high-fat food that should be avoided in most fat-reducing diets. As with other protein selections, the particular cut of pork and how it is prepared (trim visible fat; braise, roast, or broil) will make a lot of difference in the fat consumed with this item. One of the lower saturated fat selections from pork would be roasted pork tenderloin, six ounces of which would have about 8 fat grams. A broiled lean center loin is 17.8 fat grams for a similar serving size. Fat content continues to worsen if you select six ounces of roasted center rib loin with fat— you would be making a 40 fat gram selection. Pan fry that same center rib loin and you deliver a whopping 56 grams of fat to your system.

DAIRY

Dairy products should be among the least selected protein foods in your weight management program. Scientists have found consumption of dairy products to be a leading cause of atherosclerosis, heart attacks, and

"...contributors to food allergies."

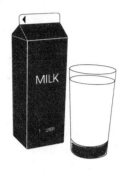

strokes. The high-fat dairy products are also those most likely to contain potentially harmful amounts of environmental contaminants including pesticide residues and hazardous radioactive substances.

This category is also among the leading contributors to food allergies. Several studies have correlated allergies to dairy products with abdominal pain, asthma, bad breath, constipation, cramps or bloating, diarrhea, eczema, gas, headaches, hives, hyperactivity, irritability, lack of energy, mental depression, muscle pain, nasal stuffiness, nutrient malabsorption, poor appetite, rashes, restlessness, runny nose, shortness of breath, and sinusitis.

Whole milk (3.7-4.0% fat) contains about 160 calories per cup, almost half of which are pure fat (80 calories fat/cup). Two-percent milk, at 120 calories per cup, has about half the fat as whole milk and perhaps may not taste as watery to some as skim milk. One-percent milk is slightly richer than skim but still only has 100 calories per cup. Therefore, when possible choose lowfat and skim milk (0-1%) and yogurts. Cultured buttermilk is about 20 percent fat. Avoid full-cream milk, cream, Half & Half, whipped toppings, and non-dairy coffee creamers (especially those made with coconut, palm, or palm kernel oil).

Most commercial frozen yogurts are high in fat, ranging from 2-7 fat grams per 4 ounce serving (if not *lowfat* or *non-fat* variety). An average medium non-fat serving contains at least seven teaspoons of sugar. When dining or preparing meals, you can substitute plain lowfat or skim yogurt for sour cream in some recipes. You can drain yogurt overnight on a coffee filter or cheesecloth-lined colander or sieve for use as a cheese spread. Also try fat-free and fruit-flavored yogurt.

Some people use lowfat or non-fat frozen yogurt in place of ice cream. This may be a good substitution, but don't forget about lowfat ice milks, sorbet, sherbet, and flavored ices. Limit regular ice cream to small servings (try a cone with one small scoop rather than a bowl with three large scoops). Avoid the rich, premium high-fat varieties.

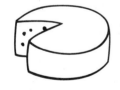

"...the sharper the cheese, the less needed for flavoring."

Cheese is a dairy product that may be tough for many people to limit or give up. Make the transition gradually, if you need to. Start with lower-fat varieties (< 2 grams butterfat per ounce) and look in recipe books for inventive ways to substitute and stretch your favorites. To prepare a dish like macaroni and cheese dish while cutting down calories and fat, add more pasta or try shredding the cheese, mix with evaporated milk and whipped egg whites, and fold in some grated Parmesan and Romano cheese. You will find you can use less cheese and still get the full flavor.

Treat cheese like eggs and only have it once or twice weekly, if at all. When you do use cheese, realize the sharper the cheese, the less needed

"Lactose intolerance... can cause bloating..."

for flavoring. Some examples of reduced- and no-fat cheeses include: lowfat and nonfat cottage cheese; 'lite' ricotta; light Swiss, Colby, or cheddar cheese; fat-free American, cheddar, or mozzarella; or hard cheese or imitation cheese made from skim milk, and dry curd. Remember that cheese substitutes without cholesterol can still be high in fat.

Lactose intolerance is a problem with dairy products that some people experience. It can cause bloating, abdominal cramping, diarrhea and other problems in someone that is *lactase-deficient*. Although many adult Caucasians have the ability to digest lactose, many Native Americans, Jews, and descendants of the Middle East, Africa, and the Orient do not.

Nursing mothers should be aware of potential problems for their babies if they consume moderate amounts of dairy products. Breast-fed babies can develop colic and other cow's milk allergy symptoms through mother's dairy consumption.

VEGETABLE PROTEIN

The well respected medical journal *Lancet* had an editorial which stated: "Formerly, vegetable proteins were classified as second-class and regarded as inferior to first-class proteins of animal origin, but this distinction has now been generally discarded." This new focus compliments the new USDA food pyramid and the new basic four food group guidelines.

Arnold Schwarzenegger, an advocate for physical fitness and bodybuilding, wrote in his bodybuilding book: "Kids nowadays...tend to go overboard [on] protein—something I believe to be totally unnecessary...[I state in] my formula for basic good eating: Eat about one gram of protein for every two pounds of body weight."

"...a lot of long term filling power..."

Unless you resorted to high levels of sugar, jellies, jams, and other essentially protein-free foods, it would be very hard to cause an appreciable loss of body protein on a mixed vegetable diet. Some advocates state we only need about 6 percent of total calories as protein (for weight maintenance). These same advocates feel it is almost impossible to get below 9 percent protein in our ordinary dietary intake.

Beans and legumes such as lentils, chick-peas, and lima beans can provide a lot of long-term *filling power* for hunger satisfaction because of their high-fiber content. This may help reduce in-between meal snacking tendencies. Complex carbohydrate foods, beans and legumes, are also high in protein, containing 170 calories (and about 1 gram fat) per 6 ounce serving. Compare this with the 480 calories and 30 fat grams in a 6 ounce broiled steak and you can see where the former can be a good choice for replacing meat.

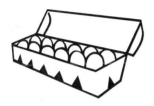

EGGS

Until lower cholesterol eggs are developed (and some have been), prudent recommendations include limiting eggs (particularly egg yolks) to no more than three per week. They should be avoided altogether if you already have elevated blood cholesterol. A chicken's egg yolk is about 80 percent fat, most of it the unhealthy saturated kind, and is one of America's most concentrated dietary sources of cholesterol. Some people can cause a 12 percent rise in blood cholesterol just by eating one egg a day. This rise in cholesterol translates into a 24 percent rise in heart attack risk. If one and a half eggs are consumed daily, this raises the risk to 32 percent.

"Interesting recipes... are as close as your local bookstore..."

Other than avoiding eggs altogether, egg substitutes (such as Egg Beaters) and egg whites are suitable. Interesting recipes substituting egg whites and other items in traditional dishes are as close as your local bookstore as more lowfat, low-cholesterol cookbooks come on the scene.

PROTEIN WRAP-UP

As we have mentioned earlier in this section, proteins come from a wide variety of food sources. Primary protein foods are fish, chicken, meat, dairy products, and legumes (dry beans and peas). Adequate protein intake, particularly when reducing weight through restricted caloric intake, helps to maintain muscle mass without excessive breakdown of lean tissue.

Current recommendations are for Americans to eat healthy by increasing their intake of fish, poultry (without the skin), and dried peas and beans. One goal could be to consume 2/3 of our protein from vegetable sources like grain, beans, and soy items. During weight maintenance, if we could reduce our protein excess from foods of animal origin (fish, meat, poultry, eggs and dairy products), we might be able to have a lower rate of heart disease than the Eskimos (high fish consumers). At the very least, we should eat only modest portions (3-4 ounces cooked) of fish, poultry, or meat. We need to shift our main eating focus (larger portion sizes) to extra vegetables, potatoes, rice, beans, and lentils.

"We need to shift our main eating focus..."

- Purchase canned fish and shellfish packed in water instead of oil.
- Select fresh fish and poultry (remove skin). Limit shrimp, lobster or sardines to no more than one serving per week.
- If you must eat veal, lamb or pork, buy ones with the least amount of visible fat.

Consumption of meat and high-fat dairy products is known to be a primary contributor to elevated risk of obesity, atherosclerosis, hypertension, stroke, and heart attack. Be an informed consumer, watching for improvements such as the specially bred cattle with extra-lean meats. In so doing, you can still occasionally enjoy this source of protein, vitamin B_6, niacin, and trace elements. Choose lean cuts of meat with little marbling.

- Beef is graded and labeled according to fat content—*Prime* being the most fat, *Choice* the next most fat, and *Select* the leanest. Purchase cuts with the least amount of visible fat and trim away excess fat. The six leanest cuts are: top round, top loin, round tip, eye of round, sirloin, and tenderloin.
- Choose ground beef labeled *Extra Lean* when available. The next best choice is *Lean*. You may also purchase some of the lean cuts listed above and have the butcher grind it for you after removing excess fat.

Select white meat turkey and chicken, extra lean ground beef, and limit goose, duck, organ meats, sausage and bacon. Ground turkey and chicken can be substituted in many ground meat dishes. Bake, broil, dry grill, or roast poultry, fish and meat instead of pan-frying or deep-fat frying. To help prevent drying and enhance flavor you may wish to baste with lemon or tomato juice, wine, or de-fatted broth.

If you decide to utilize a vegetarian diet, be sure to include nuts, soybeans, lentils, tofu, and wholegrain cereals and breads. Supplementation with lowfat milk, yogurt, cheese, and eggs (mostly egg whites) should greatly enhance nutrient intake.

Meat Eating and Resource Wasting

As a primary meat-eating country, Americans are doing several things. We are increasing our risk of many diseases, including heart attack and stroke, as well as helping to starve the rest of the world. The China-Oxford-Cornell Health Project on Nutrition, Health, and the Environment, came to the conclusion that "...whether industrialized societies...can cure themselves of their meat addictions may ultimately be a greater factor in world health than all the doctors, health insurance policies, and drugs put together."

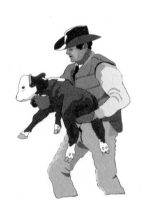

"We are... helping to starve the rest of the world."

The *majority* of harvested agricultural acreage in the United States is used to produce *livestock feed*. Less than half of the total acreage grows food for people. A given amount of land can feed *more than six times* as many people eating a vegetarian diet as those on a meat-based diet. To feed one meat eater for a year takes three-and-a-quarter acres of land. To feed one vegetarian for a year only requires one-half acre of land. It takes sixteen pounds of grain to produce one pound of feedlot beef. It takes only one pound of grain to produce a pound of bread.

It is sometimes mind-boggling how wasteful grain conversion to beef is. By transformation of our grain through livestock and into meat, we end up with only 6 percent as much food available to feed humans as we would have if they ate the grain themselves. This is certainly not *fuel efficient*.

"Millions of humans are dying needlessly..."

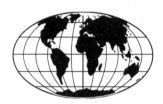

Livestock in the U.S. daily consumes enough soybeans and grain to feed more than five times the people in our country. They eat more than 80 percent of the corn and more than 95 percent of the oats we grow. If Americans could just reduce meat consumption by 10 percent, enough grain could be saved in a year to feed sixty million people—close to the estimated number of people dying from hunger-related disease each year.

In case you assumed that the majority of grain exported by our country goes to feed hungry people of the world, guess again. Two-thirds of all our grain exports goes to feed livestock rather than people. Seventy-five percent of Third World imports of oats, barley, and corn are fed to animals, not humans. Usually only a small, wealthy minority of people in most of those countries can afford meat, so some of the meat produced sometimes ends up being imported back to the United States.

The story inside the countries themselves is not much brighter. Twenty-five years ago, livestock only consumed about 6 percent of Mexico's grain. Today, it is over 50 percent and still climbing. This same trend is being repeated throughout the Third World. Where will the people of the world end up when a typical acre of Latin American land could easily produce over *twelve hundred pounds* of grain per year, yet using the same land to graze cattle barely yields *fifty pounds* of meat?

The real crime is that we absolutely *do not need* to consume as much meat and protein as we Americans do. If fact, we are hammering in our coffin nails with our appetites. Millions of humans are dying needlessly from diseases caused by meat and dairy consumption (and the associated high-fat intake), and additional millions are starving while grain is fed to livestock to produce the very food items causing so much illness and premature death.

Osteoporosis — Protein Related

"Osteoporosis is caused by several factors..."

The medical journal *Lancet* has called, "...the connection between meat-based diets and the increasing incidence of osteoporosis an *inescapable* conclusion." Osteoporosis (loss of calcium; bone thinning) is caused by several factors, one of which can be excess protein in our diets. High-protein dietary intake can lead to loss of calcium (negative calcium balance), contributing to osteoporosis.

In the United States, an average measurable bone loss by age sixty-five is:

3% *in male* **vegetarians**	**18%** *in female* **vegetarians**
7% *in male* **meat eaters**	**35%** *in female* **meat eaters**

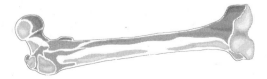

Carbohydrates $1\ gram = 4\ calories$

The technical definition of a carbohydrate is an aldehyde or ketone derivative of a polyhydric alcohol. A slightly simpler definition is a carbon containing compound (the *carbo* part) along with hydrogen and oxygen atoms generally in proportion to make water—H_2O (the *hydrate* part). How's that for a chemistry lesson? Carbohydrates are the *gasoline* of life. You may recognize them easier from this list of carbohydrates: vegetables, fruits, breads, whole-grained cereals, beans, peas, pasta, lentils and potatoes.

VEGETABLES

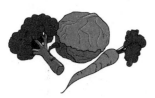

High quality (complex) carbohydrates, such as vegetables, provide many micronutrients (vitamins & minerals), water, and less calories per ounce than many convenience or snack foods. Besides being low-calorie, they tend to be lowfat (depending how they are prepared). They help to fill you up without filling you out. *Vegetables can be a wonderful staple* in any weight management program as they can be prepared and used in a variety of ways to enhance dietary appeal. Consider them for appetizers, salads, side dishes, part of main dishes, or as snacks.

"...eat a lot of vegetables."

Remember that *simple* can be better. For example, three ounces of battered and fried zucchini sticks have almost 200 calories—about 50% of which come from fat. Contrast this to the 12 calories and negligible fat in the same amount of raw zucchini.

Therefore, one key recommendation in your weight management program is to eat a lot of vegetables (raw or prepared without additional fat). Depending upon the vegetable and fiber content, it can be a dietary aid to reduce constipation and certain cancer risks.

A survey by the National Center for Health Statistics showed that on the day of the interview, almost 20% of the U.S. adult population did not eat a single vegetable. Corn and dried peas and beans, which are relatively fiber-rich, were eaten by only 20% of adults. Poor dietary choices (as mirrored in this survey) shows why the average daily fiber intake in this survey was only about 11 grams— much less than the current recommendations of 20-30 grams of daily fiber intake.

Vegetables thought to be important in cancer-risk reduction are ones high in vitamins A and C, such as dark-green leafy vegetables and yellow-orange vegetables. Almost 75% of the study group failed to have a vitamin C- or vitamin A-rich vegetable or fruit in that day's intake. Other cancer risk reducing vegetables are those in the cruciferae [or mustard] family, such as cabbage, broccoli, cauliflower, turnips, and Brussels sprouts. Less than 20% of the survey group ate any of this special family on the survey day.

BROCCOLI: Many people are not aware that this is a powerhouse of nutrition. An interesting side-light about this vegetable is that it is rich in a little-known substance called *indole carbinol*. This substance breaks down *estrogen*, a hormone which might increase the incidence of certain breast tumors. Researchers believe a cup of broccoli every other day may have enough indole carbinol to help prevent the tumors. Broccoli and certain other vegetables (e.g. carrots , spinach) also contain *beta-carotene*, a substance that may help reduce throat, lung, and bladder cancer, as well as help to reduce risk of heart attack and stroke.

As with so many other food items, be prudent in how you prepare the vegetable, such as broccoli. One cup of broccoli seasoned with cheese sauce has about 300 calories. The same broccoli seasoned with lemon juice has only 50 calories. Avoid vegetables cooked or served in butter, cream or sauce and you will tend to reduce excess calories and fats.

FRUITS

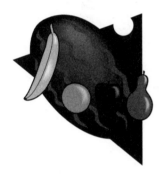

Fruits, like vegetables, tend to be low-calorie and contain fiber and micro-nutrients. They can be used for snacks, salads, appetizers, side dishes and as part of main dishes. Use fresh fruits when available and if using canned ones, try to get those packed in their own juice (not syrup) and low in sodium.

Certain fruits containing vitamins C and A are thought to reduce cancer risk too. In the Health Statistics study mentioned earlier , over 40% of the U.S. adult population had not eaten a single fruit on the day of the study.

"...fresh fruits ...less calories than dried..."

Choose a variety of fruits but do try to limit olives and avocados, especially if weight is a concern. Also be selective, even with so-called 'diet fruit platters' in restaurants. The cantaloupe balls and grapefruit sections may have about 30 calories each, but the canned pear half might have 78 calories and the canned peach, another 90. Add in the 80 calorie fruit gelatin, the 50 calorie cottage cheese and some 80 calorie dressing and you may be up to almost 440 calories in this *diet* plate. Certainly the fruit part of it is good, but don't be misled into thinking you haven't really eaten anything.

Speaking of grapefruit, scientists think *pectin* (the substance found in the peel and white membrane surrounding the citrus pulp) might lower cholesterol levels. Early studies suggest that pectin may be useful in treating clogged arteries. However, the

TABLE 11

FRESH FRUIT	FRUIT JUICE
High fiber	Very little fiber
Low calorie concentration	High calorie concentration
Longer eating time	No eating time (drink)
Satisfies hunger through bulk	Does not satisfy hunger with bulk
Sugar content slowly absorbed	Sugar content quickly absorbed
Less insulin required	More insulin required

"Avoid consuming too much fruit juice..."

amount of citrus needed to produce any beneficial results from pectin is the equivalent of about two or three grapefruit per day.

Realize that *fresh* fruits have proportionally less calories than *dried* fruits because they contain more water. However, if you snack on a few dried fruits rather than a candy bar, this is still healthier and probably saves you some calories. Even the banana (which is higher in calories than other fruits) can help in weight watching, especially considering its nutritional benefits and sweetness. Since a large one can have upwards of 120 calories or more, try to select a small or medium-sized one. You can even use it as an ice cream substitute by peeling it, wrapping it in foil, and freezing it. Slicing it into wafers, freezing them, and then eating a few of these frozen banana chips can often help satisfy a sweet-tooth.

You might want to try using fresh fruit purées instead of syrups on pancakes and French toast. If you need more sweetness, add some apple or orange juice concentrate to the purée.

Avoid consuming too much fruit juice as one glass can have the same amount of calories as several pieces of the fresh fruit, *without* the benefit of the fiber and non-water soluble micronutrients. Eating the fruit tends to be much more filling and give you a sense of eating satisfaction.

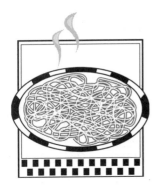

PASTA

Pasta is a complex carbohydrate that is also classified as a starch (see next subsection), but for many years it has been considered taboo for weight reducing diets. Therefore, we want to clear up some of these common misconceptions. It is a filling, low-calorie source of protein and carbohydrate that contains a lot of B-vitamins. Dried pasta (no egg) is lower in cholesterol than refrigerated pastas. Try to limit egg noodles when possible.

In general, it's not the pasta itself that is fattening, it's the things we put on top of the pasta that create the real problems. Select plain pasta instead of adding the cream, butter, or cheese sauces. If you must have sauce, use the marinara sauce instead of the Alfredo. If you need some cheese flavor, sprinkle it with Romano or Parmesan. Don't add oil to the water when cooking or butter to the steaming noodles. To limit the pasta sticking to itself, try mixing in the sauce immediately after draining. If not serving it right away, rinse the pasta with cold water and add sauce later.

STARCHES

As mentioned above, starches (like pasta) have been falsely accused of being fattening. Re-examining the problem has shown us that it is usually what goes on top of *or* in the starchy item that is the true culprit. Starches tend to be good sources of fiber, bulk, carbohydrate, protein, and vitamins.

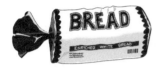

BREAD: One of many starches that used to be considered *off-limits* when reducing. The 100 calorie butter spread on the 80 calorie bread is where the fats and wasted, unhealthy majority of the 180 calorie total came from. Each meal may need to have some starch or you may stay hungry. Use enriched or whole-grain breads, bread sticks, or rolls that don't contain palm, palm kernel, or coconut oil. Acceptable choices include: corn tortillas, English muffins, Italian, or white breads, rye, pita, whole wheat, bagels made without cheese or egg, sour dough, or raisin bread without frosting. Ones to avoid are doughnuts, Danish pastry, croissants, sweet rolls, and fat-soaked toast and garlic bread. Fats can be hidden in blueberry, bran, or other muffins.

POTATOES: Avoid french-fried potatoes and regular potato salad as these tend to be prime sources of fats and unneeded calories. A large baked potato is 200 very filling calories and can give you a good source of fiber, especially if you eat the peel. Avoid the butter, sour cream, cheese, and bacon bits you might ordinarily add to it. For moistness and flavor, try using lowfat milk to mash the potato in the peel or use a sauce made with tamari, olive oil, and lemon juice. You might also try topping the potato with steamed vegetables, salsa, steak sauce, mustard or horseradish for flavor variations. Occasionally, eat the yellow-skin potatoes plain and enjoy their natural goodness (some find them more flavorful than the white varieties).

"A large baked potato is 200 very filling calories..."

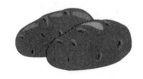

Sweet potatoes may sound fattening, but actually contain no more calories than white potatoes. A four-ounce serving has some vitamin C and fiber, more potassium than a banana, and a lot of beta-carotene. They are good plain baked also.

Instant potatoes shouldn't be considered a diet food. As is true with many processed foods, they tend to be high in sodium and preservatives, and not nearly as filling as a regular baked potato. Many mixes contain fat or require you to add oil or butter, thus increasing calorie and fat intake.

CEREALS: Choose low-sugar hot or cold cereals as most are low in fat with little, if any, cholesterol. Avoid the granola-type cereals that contain coconut or other hydrogenated oils. Cereals containing seeds and nuts may have a higher fat content than all-grain brands but can fall within your daily fat allotment. Whole-grain cereals are a good source of fiber and may help reduce constipation and might lower serum cholesterol. More than 80% of adults in the Health Statistic survey did not consume any high-fiber cereal on the interview day.

Flaxseed is a cereal grain (used mainly in Europe and Canada) containing a type of fatty acid, *linolenic acid*, similar to that found in fish oil. This substance might inhibit the body's production of prostaglandins, hormone-like substances that may contribute to the formation of tumors. It may also be of benefit in certain conditions such as asthma, arthritis, and psoriasis.

CRACKERS: Select lowfat crackers when possible and avoid butter or cheese crackers. Acceptable choices would be zwieback, graham, rye crispbreads, bread sticks, matzo, melba toast, and fat-free soda crackers. Remember that these calories add up too. One melba toast has about 20 calories and two saltines have about 25 calories.

SUGARS

As part of the body's digestive process, carbohydrates are usually broken down into both simple and complex sugars (and of course we can eat plain, simple sugars also). A big problem with simple sugar ingestion is that it provides only empty calories. An empty calorie is one that essentially supplies none of the nutrients needed by the body for health maintenance— no vitamins, minerals, or enzymes. Under certain conditions, sugars along with complex carbohydrates may stimulate overeating and obesity.

"Sugars are often disguised..."

We should therefore limit simple and refined sugar products and increase our consumption of higher quality carbohydrates (some of which have already been mentioned). Simple sugars are found in items such as soft drinks, jams, cakes, fruit drinks, donuts, ice cream, table sugar, honey, cookies, and chocolate. It takes a lot of simple sugars before you are *filled up*. Think of them as the drugs and processed chemicals they really are. We consume between 130-150 pounds of sugar per person per year.

These sugars are *physically* and *psychologically* addicting— the more you eat, the more you want to eat. The more simple carbohydrates you eat, the faster they are burned. Dramatic fluctuations in blood sugar levels can eventually lead to anxiety or depression. Children also have greater hormonal response to refined sweeteners than do adults.

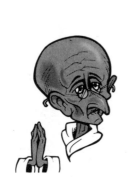

As health-seeking adults, we need to be the examples for our children. This point is driven home in the story about Mahatma Gandhi, the great Indian leader. It is reported that a mother had taken her young son to the sage and asked him to instruct the lad to stop eating sugar. Gandhi told her, "Come back in a week." Puzzled, the woman left, returning with her son after the requested interval. Gandhi then followed through with the woman's original request, instructing the youngster to avoid sugar. After he had finished, the mother asked Gandhi why he had postponed the matter for a week. "Oh," he replied, "first I had to give up sugar."

Be on guard against unhealthy products that advertise themselves to be sugar-free. Sugars are often disguised by calling them by their real names. Read labels for ingredients ending in **tol** or **ose**, such as sorbitol (sugarless gums), mannitol, maltose, lactose, dextrose (simple sugar), fructose (fruit sugar), glucose, or sucrose (cane sugar). Other ways of describing sugar products are by calling them corn or high-fructose corn syrup, honey, brown sugar, molasses, and natural sweeteners. These might be slight improvements over sugar, but they still consist of empty calories and very little nutrients, if any. Obesity, wide fluctuations in blood sugar, and tooth decay can still be caused by these sweeteners. Used *in moderation*, artificially sweetened foods and beverages are considered okay.

FACT or FICTION: Sugar-free/sugarless products can contain sweeteners that are just as high in calories as table sugar.

FACT! These products often contain high calorie sweeteners including honey, corn syrup, mannitol, fructose, or sorbitol.

Beware of chocolate substitutes, like carob, which are sometimes no better than the chocolate itself. Carob candy contains saturated fat, sometimes more than a Hershey bar. White chocolate has about the same amount of *calories and fat* as chocolate or carob.

Read labels. A tablespoon of ketchup contains a teaspoon of sugar. Frozen yogurt has 135-150 calories per one-half cup; supermarket-style ice cream has less (but more fat).

COMPLEX CARBOHYDRATES

"...complex carbohydrates should be our largest dietary intake..."

Complex carbohydrates include many of the items we have already mentioned like bread, cereal, pasta, and potatoes. These items add fiber, vitamins, and minerals to our diets. They are also important as substrates (food) for our brain cells and nerve tissue. High quality carbohydrates help spare muscle and other body proteins when restricting calories (e.g. weight loss attempts), especially before the fat stores can be broken down. Approximately 100 grams (400 calories) of carbohydrate per day is needed to spare protein and avoid large weight shifts due to water (fluid) fluctuation.

For healthy weight management, whether losing or maintaining, complex carbohydrates should be our largest dietary intake from all the food groups. A generally accepted percentage would be 50-60% or more of calories we consume. Ounce for ounce, they tend to be more filling and most have fewer calories than most meats and cheeses.

BEANS/LEGUMES

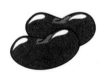

Legumes such as lima beans, chick-peas, and lentils provide long-term eating satisfaction because of their high-fiber. Containing about 8 to 9 grams of fiber per cup (cooked), they are second only to wheat bran as a source of fiber.

Potassium, calcium, iron, zinc, and B vitamins are also provided by these dietary selections. They are also high in protein and have no cholesterol and little fat (except soybeans which are high in unsaturated fat), which makes them an excellent meat replacement in a varied diet. One cup of cooked dried peas or beans contains only about 200 to 300 calories—certainly sensible in any weight management program.

Beware of processed beans, such as refried beans, as they probably contain a lot of lard. If needed, you may wish to purchase vegetarian refried beans which are free of lard.

If *gas* production by beans is a problem, it can be reduced in several ways. One is through the use of a commercial product called *BEANO*. A few drops added to the beans greatly reduces the gas problem. Another method is to soak the beans and discard the water, or partially cook the beans, discard the water, and use fresh water to continue cooking (though this gets rid of some of

"Carbohydrates are very filling."

the water-soluble vitamins). Still another method might be to add about one-half to one teaspoon of baking soda to the water when cooking. Some beans, such as lentils, limas, chick peas, and white beans also tend to produce less gaseous problems than others. Try not to consume additional quantities of *gas-producing* vegetables in your diet at the same time you are adding the beans.

SOYBEANS: Utilized in abundance in Asian cuisine. They can be canned, boiled, or processed as bean curd (tofu). *Lecithin*, abundant in soybeans, might assist prevention of alcoholic cirrhosis of the liver. Liver cancer in animals has been shown to be prevented by isoflavones in the beans. The isoflavones are thought to break down the toxic substances that can cause the malignancy. Exercise caution in utilizing this food product though; it also contains protease inhibitors which have been linked to the development of pancreatic cancer.

BULK/FIBER

Carbohydrates are very filling. Consider how filling vegetables, fruits, bread, potatoes, pasta, and rice can be. They are good sources of energy because our bodies are quite efficient at burning them. Remember fiber and bulking agents help to promote bowel regularity.

"Fiber refers to ...roughage."

They also contain less than half the calories fats contain (gram per gram), so you are unlikely to overeat and gain too much excess weight by switching to a high carbohydrate diet. The bulk alone might slow you down. Consider eating 990 calories of air-popped popcorn. That would require you to eat *33 cups*. Compare this to the one large chocolate milkshake that you've had in the past for the *same* 990 calories.

You can eat a lot of carbohydrates for relatively few calories. The same does not hold true for fats or chocolate candy bars. When you have had a little fat (or chocolate), you have had a lot of calories. The healthier, behavior changing path is to replace fats with filling, fiber-rich carbohydrates such as vegetables, fruits, and whole grains.

Realize that some healthy sounding foods can be loaded with fat, calories, and/or cholesterol. Many deli or bakery bran muffins have far more eggs, sugar, and hydrogenated oil than they do oat or wheat bran.

Fiber & Constipation

Fiber refers to the indigestible part of plant foods, sometimes known as roughage. It is not found in foods of animal origin (e.g. dairy products, meat). Fiber has been found to inhibit the absorption of carbohydrates and fats, sometimes even helping to lower blood cholesterol. Fibers are further classified into two groups based on their water solubility. Both types are of benefit.

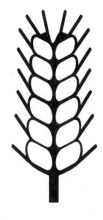

(a) ***Insoluble fibers*** are part of the structural components of plant cell walls and include lignin, hemicelluloses, and cellulose. They create soft bulk by absorbing many times their own weight of water (called *bulk-forming ability*) and also decrease elimination time through the intestines. They produce more frequent bowel movements (enhance regularity) with softer stools, and may help prevent and even treat uncomplicated forms of constipation, hemorrhoids, and diverticulosis. Colon cancer risk may also be lowered by the diluting effect of the fiber on potentially harmful substances in the intestine. The best sources of insoluble fibers are seeds, nuts, peas, dried beans, whole-wheat bread and cereals, rice bran, corn bran, wheat bran, and the skins of vegetables and fruits. Of note is that rice bran has been found to lower blood cholesterol and wheat bran may reduce breast cancer risk through lowering of estrogen levels.

(b) ***Soluble fibers*** are usually within the plant cells themselves and include mucilages, gums, and pectin. These fibers produce a gel (when in the presence of fluid) which slows stomach emptying and sugar absorption from the intestines (improving glucose tolerance). Diabetics can especially benefit from this action as blood sugar levels tend to be more controlled, which in turn may reduce insulin requirements. Primary sources of soluble fibers are dried beans and peas, oat bran, rice bran, barley, flax seed, psyllium, fruits and vegetables. The first four, oat bran, rice bran, dried peas and beans, have been shown to lower cholesterol by their binding action on bile acids.

"Most Americans don't eat enough fiber..."

It has been shown that fiber-rich foods usually *enhance the nutrient content* of the whole diet, particularly if they take the place of high-fat items. Whole-wheat bread, potatoes, and fresh fruits and vegetables have few calories for their bulk (as they are lowfat). By providing bulk, they slow stomach emptying, give a full feeling, and satisfy appetite much quicker than low- or no-fiber foods. The stomach-brain axis needs about twenty minutes to register a feeling of eating satisfaction, so the extra chewing time bulky, high-fiber items take contributes to this satiety. This is something important in controlling weight, as is the slower emptying of the stomach and the feeling of fullness fiber provides.

Foods and drinks with minimal or no fiber tend to have higher calorie concentrations and require little or no chewing. Moderate amounts of these types of foods (e.g. candy, sugar, fats, fruit juices, alcohol, soft drinks, etc.) can be ingested before appetite is satisfied. For example, one large orange might reduce our appetite, whereas the orange juice containing approximately the sugar and calories of 3 oranges might not. *Lack of dietary fiber* has been linked with appendicitis, colon cancer, constipation, coronary heart disease, diabetes, diverticular disease, gallbladder disease, hemorrhoids, irritable bowel syndrome, and varicose veins.

Most Americans don't eat enough fiber— averaging between 11 and 15 grams per day. The National Cancer Institute recommends an intake of at least 25-35 grams a day. This amount should help promote bowel motility and reduce constipation, something prevalent on many *diets*. A working definition of constipation would be a failure to have a bowel movement at least every second day (though this will vary from individual to individual), and without straining or pain. The stool tends to be small, narrow, and very firm.

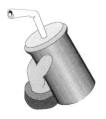

A primary cause of constipation is lack of fiber in the diet. Other things which might contribute include certain medications (e.g. tranquilizers, antidepressants, antacids), gastro-intestinal problems, stress, insufficient exercise, or too little fluid intake. A healthy recommendation is to talk to your doctor about this problem, especially if there is a recent change in bowel habits during mid-life or later. The following list will contain suggestions to increase dietary fiber, which should be beneficial for all the reasons already mentioned:

"Drink adequate fluid daily..."

- Eat high-fiber breakfast cereals (oatmeal, bran-based and other whole-grain cereals, etc.) as breakfast should be an important supplier of daily fiber. Unprocessed wheat bran (1-2 tbsp), seeds, chopped nuts, or dried fruits can be added to cereals and muffin or pancake batters if needed and if *not* attempting weight reduction. Wheat bran or rice bran can also be added to cakes, cookies, desserts, yogurt, casseroles, and soups. If you are unable to tolerate bran, you might wish to try psyllium-based fiber supplements.
- Bran does not always mean best. A survey found some commercial oat bran muffins containing almost 30 grams of fat. One had over 800 calories.
- Drink adequate fluid daily (at least 6 to 8 glasses) since fiber works like a sponge, absorbing many times its own weight of fluid. Don't forget to increase your fluid intake when increasing dietary fiber or else you can actually *cause* severe constipation to occur.
- Use bran-enriched or whole-wheat bread, rolls or bread sticks that do not contain coconut, palm, or palm kernel oil. It would take 3 slices of white bread to have as much fiber as 1 slice of whole-wheat bread.
- Eat fresh fruit with edible skins instead of just consuming fruit juice. Fresh is preferred over canned, peeled, and juiced (puréed) fruit.
- Consume more vegetables, salads, and legumes—especially dried beans, lentils, baked beans, broccoli, avocado, potatoes with skins, Brussels sprouts, carrots, celery, cabbage, and peas. Fresh vegetables have more fiber and vitamins than canned or frozen ones. Some good selections might include peas, spinach, turnips, broccoli, cabbage, etc. Gram for gram, lima, pinto, or kidney beans have almost twice the amount of fiber as green beans. Eat vegetables raw or slightly steamed. Whole vegetables are preferable to juiced (puréed) vegetables as they have more fiber and vitamins (some vitamins are not water-soluble and aren't present in the juice).
- Enjoy brown, long-grained, whole rice. This is not the same as the *fried-rice* you ate at the Chinese restaurant.
- Use whole-wheat flour in place of white flour in cooking and baking, even in pastas. Whole-grain products tend to retain more of the vitamins and fiber essential in a healthy diet than do refined-grain items.

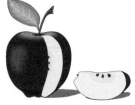

"...quick introduction of fiber can cause problems..."

- Snack on fresh or dried high-fiber fruits (e.g. prunes, dates, apples, or raspberries), popcorn, nuts or seeds, whole-wheat crackers, carrot or celery sticks, and high-fiber bars (lowfat). Raspberries have four times as much fiber as cherries. Limit amounts of some of the higher calorie items if you need to manage your weight.
- Exercise regularly as this tends to help with bowel regularity due to stronger and healthier abdominal muscles and better bowel motility.
- Avoid taking harsh laxatives frequently for constipation as your intestines may build up a dependence upon these and actually require them for bowel motility. Consult your physician for advice.

In the second National Health and Nutrition Examination Survey, over 80% of those interviewed had not eaten any high-fiber cereals or whole-grain breads; over 40% hadn't eaten a single fruit; and over 20% did not eat a vegetable on the day of the interview. High-fiber items, such as dried peas and beans or corn, had only been eaten by 20% of adults that day as well, which meant that the average fiber intake for most respondents was about one-half of current recommendations.

Not all foods high in complex carbohydrates are high in fiber. Whole wheat bread or brown rice are higher in fiber (as well as being complex carbohydrates) than white bread and white rice.

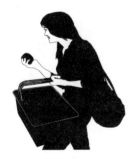

High fiber foods should be added to dietary intake slowly, as quick introduction of fiber can cause problems (such as diarrhea, bloating, and flatulence). This is a case where *small changes* over a reasonable period of time is prudent.

One could go a long way towards improving the American intake of fiber and decreasing many health risks by becoming a semi-vegetarian. This is someone who eats the majority of their dietary intake as grains, vegetables, fruit, legumes, and lowfat dairy products with occasional supplementation of fish, poultry, and beef.

A recent newcomer on the fiber scene is soy fiber from the inside of the soybean hull (not to be confused with soy bran). It has a nutty smell and taste, is a more concentrated source of fiber than oat bran, and may prove to reduce blood cholesterol in those with cholesterol elevations. One additional benefit is that it contains soluble as well as insoluble fiber.

Although fiber can be beneficial, *too much fiber can cause problems too*. Fiber is known to bind some vitamins and minerals, preventing their uptake and increasing their elimination through the bowel. Vitamin B_{12} and minerals such as iron, copper, zinc, calcium, phosphorus, and magnesium can be bound by excessive fiber.

Eat *at least* several servings of vegetables and fruits *daily*. In **table 12** (following page), LOW fiber items contain 1 gram of fiber per listed serving. MEDIUM fiber items have 1 to 3 grams of fiber. HIGH fiber items have 3 grams of fiber per amounts listed.

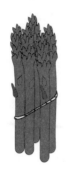

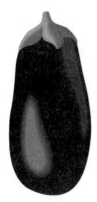

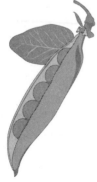

TABLE 12

Fiber Content * of Food

LOW FIBER

Vegetables:	asparagus (4)	celery (1 stalk)	green pepper (2 rings)
	mushrooms (1/2 cup)	radishes (10)	onion (1/2 cup)
Fruits:	grapefruit (1/2)	grapes (12)	lemon (1 slice)
	orange, mandarin (1/2 cup)	pineapple (1/2 cup)	plums (2 med.)

MEDIUM FIBER

Vegetables:	avocado (1/2)	bean sprouts (1/2 cup)	Brussels sprouts (1/2 cup)
	cabbage (1/2 cup)	cauliflower (1/2 cup)	coleslaw (1/2 cup)
	eggplant (1/2 cup)	green beans (1/2 cup)	lettuce (1 cup)
	okra (1/2 cup)	dill pickle (1/2 cup)	tomato (1)
	tomato sauce (1/2 cup)		
Fruits:	applesauce (1/2 cup)	apricot (2)	banana (1/2)
	cantaloupe (1/2)	sweet cherries (10)	fig (1)
	fruit salad (1/2 cup)	honeydew (1/8)	nectarine (1)
	olives (10)	orange (1)	peach (1)
	pear (1)	raisins (2 Tbsp.)	rhubarb (1/2 cup)
	strawberries (1/2 cup)	tangerine (1)	

HIGH FIBER

Vegetables:	broccoli (1/2 cup)	peas (1/2 cup)	sauerkraut (1/2 cup)
	spinach (1/2 cup)	turnips (1/2 cup)	
Fruits:	apple & peel (3")	dried dates (5)	stewed prunes (1/2 cup)
	raspberries (1/2 cup)	*Adapted from 'Composition of Food' by McCance and Widdowson.*	

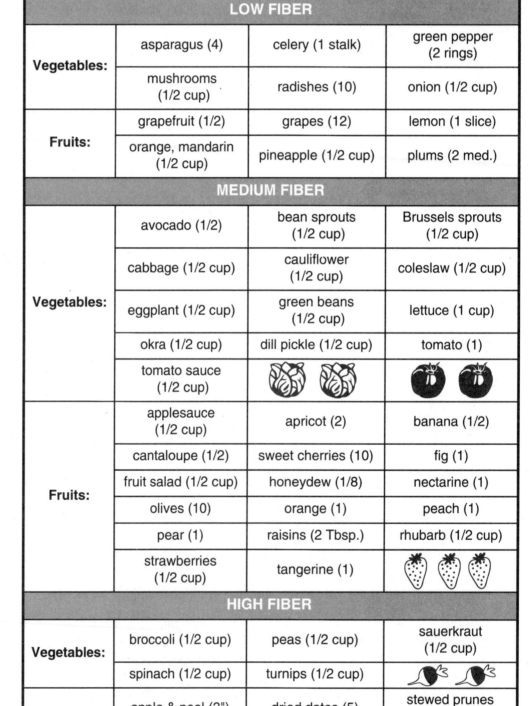

Fats

1 gram = 9 calories

Fat is found in many foods of plant and animal origin and is an essential portion of our dietary needs. *Triglycerides* comprise about 98% of dietary fats consumed. Fat is a major storehouse of internal energy (being twice as many calories per gram as protein or carbohydrate), and a carrier of the important fat-soluble vitamins: A, D, E, and K. It also imparts taste and palatability to foods. In humans, it is essential in manufacturing antibodies, it cushions the skin and joints, insulates against cold, and protects internal organs.

Essential fatty acids (e.g. linoleic acid) which are necessary for healthy skin and proper growth are also supplied by dietary fat. These fatty acids are the basic chemical units of fat and can be classified (depending upon how many hydrogen atoms they contain) as either saturated, mono-unsaturated, or polyunsaturated. Dietary fats we consume are variable mixtures of these three types of fatty acids.

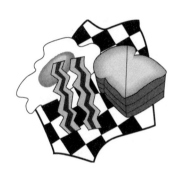

Saturated fatty acids: Highest amounts generally found in foods of *animal origin* (meats and processed meats, poultry—skin and fat, eggs and dairy products) but *also in* certain vegetable oils, such as coconut, palm and palm kernel oils. These fatty acids tend to be *solid* at room temperature and raise blood cholesterol levels as much as dietary intake of cholesterol. In fact, saturated fats are *twice as effective at raising* blood cholesterol as polyunsaturated fats are in lowering it. Chocolate contains lots of saturated fat. The darker and more bitter the chocolate, the more fat it contains. Milk chocolate has about 56 percent of its calories from fat (34% from saturated fat); bittersweet gets almost 93 percent of calories from fat (56% from saturated fat).

Mono-unsaturated fatty acids: Found in *both* plant and animal fats. Vegetable shortening, some margarines, and oils from avocados, olives, and peanuts tend to be high in these fatty acids.

Polyunsaturated fatty acids: Fats *usually from plants*. Large suppliers would be cottonseed, soybean, corn, sunflower, and safflower oils. Also found in some fish and shellfish. These tend to be *liquid* at room temperature and lower blood cholesterol.

"Chocolate contains lots of saturated fat."

Excessive calorie intake is not always the problem in weight management. The biggest culprit tends to be excessive calories from fats. Some studies have shown that dietary fat reduction can help maintain weight loss with fewer fluctuations than more traditional calorie-counting programs. Your body handles 2000 calories from pizza and fried foods much differently than 2000 calories from fruits and vegetables. Fat calories are fattening because almost all (97-98%) of the fat eaten goes straight to the body's fat cells for unlimited storage. Fat has more than twice the calories per gram as carbohydrates and proteins.

Similar people eating identical calories but with different proportions from fats will lose weight at different rates. The diet *higher in fat* will generally lead to *greater*

"Nuts, seeds, and all oils are also high in fats."

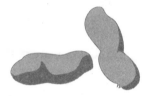

fat accumulation on the individual and a slower weight loss than the lower fat participant. Fats in our diets require less energy to be converted into body fat than do dietary proteins and carbohydrates. Thus a lowfat diet is best for weight management.

Average Americans consume 40-50% of their dietary intake as fat. Just reducing daily fat intake can save a huge amount of wasted calories because excess body fat tends to be associated with excess fat intake. The body only requires about 5% fat content in the diet. In order to lose weight (and body fat), an intake of 10-20% total dietary fat is recommended. The American Heart Association recommends that fats should not exceed 30% of daily caloric intake, with 10% of calories from saturated fatty acids, and not more than 10% from polyunsaturated fatty acids, with the rest being mono-unsaturated fatty acids.

Even though people may be eating more margarine over butter and drinking skim milk over whole milk, they're *also consuming more* packaged foods, fast foods, processed meats, cheese, and frozen desserts— all food products tending to be high in fat. The National Frozen Pizza Institute states that we consume 1.8 billion slices of frozen pizza annually.

Nuts, seeds, and all oils are also high in fat. Many physiologic associations have been identified with dietary fat intake, particularly excessive amounts that are typical of Americans. Some of these include:
- atherosclerosis
- cancer (colon, breast, prostate, and endometrium), diabetes, hypertension, stroke, and heart disease risks lower with fat at 10-15% levels, and with low dietary cholesterol
- coronary diseases
- estrogen levels lowered in blood (with reduced amount of dietary fat)
- gallstones
- obesity, overweight

Intake of 33.5% fat increases risk of heart disease and cancer ten times that of more moderate intake.

Since *Americans talk thin and eat fat*, here are some tips to help reduce dietary fat intake:

"Eat high-fat foods in smaller portions..."

- Foods containing less than 30% fat, such as cereal products, beans, breads, vegetables, and fruits, should be more prominent in the diet.
- Plan meals using substitutions and modifications. Eat high-fat foods in smaller portions and less often. Try to gradually eliminate these foods altogether and substitute lowfat food in their place.
- Remove skin from chicken and turkey before cooking. Select white meat over dark meat.
- Reduce whole egg usage and substitute egg whites or Egg Beaters.
- Eat less meat and fewer dairy products. Avoid whole milk and whole milk products. Use lowfat or nonfat dairy products, such as skim milk and low- or non-fat cheeses, when possible.

- Avoid red meats loaded with saturated fat, such as luncheon meats, bacon, and sausage. If you do eat red meat, choose lean cuts with little marbling and trim all visible fat. Trimming all visible fat before broiling can cut the fat by almost 20 percent. Try eating smaller portions (four to five ounces). Choose extra lean ground beef.
- Use marinades for lowfat meats to make them tender and more flavorful. Quick and easy marinades can be made from onion soup, beef broth, tomato soup, or red wine vinegar mixed with Worcestershire sauce and minced garlic.
- Eat fish, chicken, and turkey when possible.
- Cook skinless chicken breasts in a hot skillet sprayed with a little non-stick vegetable coating. Even without flouring or batter, the flavor can be close to *regular fried* chicken.
- Avoid high cholesterol foods, such as organ meats (e.g. liver).
- Use fat-free cooking methods. Broil, braise, roast, barbecue, microwave or bake but never fry anything (markedly limit fried foods). When we make or eat french fries or potato chips, we turn the original vegetable into a vehicle for fat and salt.

"Use fat-free cooking methods."

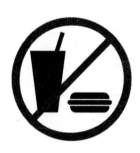

- De-fat meat drippings and broths before using. Use a long-handled spoon, metal skimmer, or bulb baster to skim the fat from soups, sauces, and gravies. An inexpensive plastic gravy separator (that drains from the bottom of the cup) may be a good lowfat investment.
- Floating a paper towel on top of hot soup can help absorb fat or it can be folded and used as a blotter to dab off the excess fat. Try to prepare soups, sauces, and gravies early enough to refrigerate them, which will allow the fat to congeal and rise to the top for removal. Even canned stock can be refrigerated.
- Sauté onions and other vegetables with minimal oil or even water.
- Steam vegetables in a little water and add herbs and lemon juice instead adding butter.
- Use vegetable spreads, tomato sauces, or mustards rather than butter, margarine, mayonnaise, or fatty gravies.
- If your sauce or soup has fat floating in it, quickly dip an ice cube into the hot liquid to solidify the excess fat on the surface to make removal easier.
- Use minimal amounts of all types of oil and fats— all are high calorie. Avoid coconut oil and hydrogenated palm oil foodstuffs.
- Use low-calorie salad dressing. Limit mayonnaise and oil dressings. Most commercial salad dressings, whether creamy or oily, get 90 percent of their calories from fat. Choose low- or no-oil dressings. Try making your own salad dressing with a low- or no-fat yogurt base or cottage cheese that is whipped in the blender.
- Avoid or limit high-fat fast foods, cookies, nuts, cakes, ice cream, pastries, granola, crackers, and chip dips.
- Acceptable lowfat sauces and seasonings have 1 gram of fat or less per serving.
- Select seasoned vinegar, herb/spice blends, or lemon juice without added salt for dressings.
- Tomato or wine-based sauces are typically lower in fat than those made from butter, sour cream, cheese, eggs, or cream.

"...whole milk ads should say 50% fat."

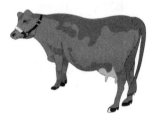

- Choose fat-reduced polyunsaturated or canola margarines. Use polyunsaturated oils or mono-unsaturated oils (e.g. olive, Canola) in moderation.
- Have meatless entrees occasionally. Substitute legumes or grains for meat in some meals. Avoid excessive nuts, oils, creams, or cheese in the dishes. Some meatless dishes (e.g. quiche) have more fat than meat.
- Mashed potatoes can be whipped with skim milk, plain yogurt, lowfat buttermilk, or chicken broth instead of using whole milk and butter.
- Plan ahead so you don't get talked into pot luck in meal choices.
- When using oils, select the following: canola, cottonseed, olive, partially hydrogenated soybean, corn, sunflower, and safflower oil.

The percentage of fat listed for milk is shown as a percentage of the milk's weight (i.e. % fat per weight, not per calories). Milk is mostly water, so the percentage contributed by fat to the total weight is small. It is more meaningful to look at the percentage of milk's calories that come from fat.

When available, select lowfat and skim milk (0-1%). One-percent milk has a slightly richer taste than skim and contains about 100 calories a cup. Two-percent milk has less of a watery taste to many than skim, contains about half the fat as whole milk and has 120 calories a cup. Whole milk (3.7% fat) has 160 calories a cup, with half the calories as pure fat (80 calories fat a cup). The whole milk ads should say 50% fat. Because of this, some authorities feel children over the age of two should consume only skim milk.

TABLE 13

Milk Type	Calories 1 cup	% Calories from FAT	Fat Grams	Cholesterol mg.
Whole milk	150	48%	8	34
Lowfat (2%)	121	35%	4.7	18
Lowfat (1%)	102	23%	2.6	10
Skim milk	86	4%	0.4	4

BUTTER/MARGARINE: You might have believed margarine to be a healthier choice than butter. One tablespoon of butter has 64 calories of saturated fat, while the same amount of margarine has 20 saturated fat calories. However, they are both 100% fat and each have 100 calories per tablespoon (35 per pat). Therefore, margarine is *just as fattening* as butter (though slightly more heart friendly) and needs to be reduced or omitted when possible. If you still utilize them, the best margarines are those listing liquid oil as the first ingredient.

THE 30% SOLUTION: Some weight managers expound the use of a 30% rule when watching fat intake. Since the American Heart Association has recommended limiting fats to no more than 30% of daily intake, this begins to have some practical validity. This 30% solution advocates making foods containing 30% or less fat a prominent part of the diet. Their theory is that these foods are readily burned off and metabolized (since they contain more protein and carbohydrates than fat), and that foods over 30% (particularly over 40%) are mostly stored in our body's fat and very difficult to metabolize.

An easy way to roughly evaluate the fat content of a food is to multiply the grams of fat by 9 (or 10 if you want a ballpark figure). If the result totals more than a third of the food's calories, that food is considered high in fat.

Other advocates point out that just limiting ourselves to foods under 30% fat may make us miss out on other beneficial aspects of food variety. They mention that some higher fat foods (such as seeds, nuts, and avocados) are nutritious and can even help lower blood cholesterol. Their motto is that *moderation, not elimination,* is the goal.

HIDDEN FAT: Watch out for those 91% *fat-free* deli meats. They may be reporting percent *fat by weight,* not by calories. Some supposedly *diet* dinners can contain 20 grams or more of fat per dinner. Don't just rely on your taste buds to help you detect fat as many times it is hidden by other flavors and textures in the food. For example, look at the grams of fat in the following items:

- Cheesecake 4 oz—22 fat grams
- Chicken nuggets (6)—15.4 fat grams
- Fast food taco or tostada—11 fat grams
- Mayonnaise 1 tbsp.—11 fat grams
- McD.L.T.—37 fat grams

- McLean burger—10 fat grams
- Potato chips (10)—7 fat grams (almost 3/4 gram fat per chip!)
- Seafood calamari rings—21 fat grams

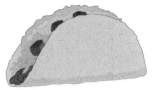

"...fats...can go by many names."

A fast food quarter-pound cheeseburger and regular order of fries contains about 41 fat grams. This can almost use the U.S. daily recommendation of fat grams in one meal.

Coffee whiteners are another hidden source of fat many people don't think about. One tablespoon of powdered creamer is 3 fat grams (mostly saturated fat). Switch to skim milk for fat savings.

When reading labels for fats, realize they can go by many names. A few of the more common ones are vegetable oil, palm and palm kernel oil, soybean oil, partially hydrogenated vegetable oil, and cocoa butter.

REDUCING WEIGHT: Excess calories are stored as body fat, period. This is true whether they come from fats, proteins, or carbohydrates. However, as already mentioned, calories consumed from fats are stored in fat cells more readily.

To maintain weight, calories taken in through food should balance those used by the body. You will gain weight if you eat more fat than you burn and will lose weight if you metabolize more fat than you consume. If reducing weight, more calories should be used than taken in.

In general you need a deficit of 3,500 calories to lose one pound of body fat. If you have a 500 calorie a day deficit (through eating less and/or being more active), this would accomplish this 3,500 calorie deficit in one week.

Permanent weight loss is a gradual process that can require months to achieve but is certainly worthwhile. Reducing the fat in our dietary intake is a great place to start.

The following example illustrates the power of the concept of simple trade-offs.

	Calories	% Fat
2 plain yeast donuts -or-	352	57%
2 pieces whole wheat toast +		
1 tsp. jelly on each	150	13%

Making this substitution 5 days a week may make a difference of 15 pounds of fat in one year!

Animal Products

As has been mentioned in several sections, food from animals tends to be *higher in saturated fats* and increases dietary risks in several areas. The more animal protein some populations consume, the higher their rates of many forms of cancer, diabetes, heart disease, gallstones, stroke, kidney stones and other kidney related diseases.

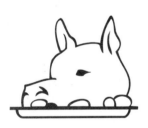

Data from the China-Oxford-Cornell Study showed that populations deriving 70% of their protein from animal products (like typical Americans) have *significant* health problems compared to populations consuming 5% of their protein from animal sources. They have *seventeen times* the death rate from heart disease, and the women are five times more likely to die from breast cancer.

The more red meat and animal fat one eats, the higher the risk of cancer of the colon. The problem with half the calories of whole milk being from fats has been mentioned previously. Since dairy products are inherently high in fat and protein, they are contributors to the cancer, heart, obesity, and other health risks associated with various animal products. If one wishes to reduce fat intake to 20% or less, you almost have to give up food from animals altogether.

"Cholesterol... found in foods of animal origin..."

Cholesterol

Cholesterol is a white, waxy, fat-like material found in foods of animal origin but not from plants. It comprises the structure of our cell membranes; is a building block for our skin's vitamin D production; and is a component in bile acids, adrenal and sex hormones. It is essential to life and is manufactured by the body (mostly in our liver) so that we are not dependent upon cholesterol in our diets to meet our needs.

"...most significant problem ...fat in our diets..."

Our body makes 800-1500 mg each day, depending upon our dietary amount. Animal foods typically provide 300-600 mg cholesterol per day.

The amount produced by our bodies is influenced by the amount of cholesterol in the foods we eat, but the most significant problem seems to be the fat in our diets (particularly saturated fats). Since hereditary elevations are seen in only a small number of people, you should be aware of the following *dietary factors* affecting blood cholesterol level (**BCL**):

- **Fats and Oils:** Fat *amount* and *type* has a greater affect on BCL than dietary cholesterol. Saturated fats (meat & dairy products) tend to raise cholesterol levels by somehow interfering with the ability of the liver to eliminate excess cholesterol. Mono- and polyunsaturated fats (avocados, olives, nuts, seeds & their oils, and fish oils) tend to lower BCL and/or other fats in the blood. Mono-unsaturated fats don't lower BCL as much as polyunsaturated fats do, but they do lower the *bad* (LDL) cholesterol. Polyunsaturated fats reduce harmful LDL but may also lower helpful (HDL) levels. Omega-3 fatty acid found in fish intake may raise HDL and lower LDL and triglyceride levels.

- **Cholesterol in food:** Its affect on BCL depends upon the person, as well as the types of fats and fiber consumed during the same meal. Even though not all foods containing cholesterol raise the BCL (e.g. yogurt, fish), it is recommended cholesterol intake be limited to 100 mg per 1000 calories—not to exceed 300 mg per day (the amount in one egg yolk). Even if no cholesterol is ingested, BCL can rise if the meal has a lot of *saturated fat*.

"HDL is known to remove cholesterol from body tissues."

- **Fiber:** The soluble fiber found in fruits (fruit pectins), vegetables, oat bran (due to its content of oat gum), psyllium, and dried beans and peas (legumes, chick peas, navy beans, pinto beans) can help to lower BCL. Another helpful source of soluble fiber is gum (like guar gum found in dried peas and seeds and stems of tropical plants). Soluble fibers tend to reduce LDL (bad) cholesterol while maintaining HDL (good) cholesterol. Other items such as nuts, seeds, and rice bran can also be of benefit.

Cholesterol and fat are transported in our blood combined with proteins, forming complexes called *lipoproteins*. Two of these complexes are known as high-density (HDL) and low-density (LDL) lipoproteins. HDL is known to remove cholesterol from body tissues. LDL tends to deposit cholesterol on the walls of arteries, especially when you have a surplus of cholesterol in the blood stream. These deposits are irritating and cause damage to the linings of the arteries. The body then produces plaque in these arteries in an attempt to repair them. However, depending upon time and amount of injury, too much plaque may be built, which in turn can block blood flow. Depending upon the location and amount of blockage, this can lead to kidney failure, impotence, circulatory problems, blindness, stroke, heart disease or heart attack.

The National Institutes of Health consensus panel recommends a blood cholesterol level of less than 180 mg/dL if under 30 years of age. If older, 200 mg/dL is the upper limit recommended. For each 1% elevation in blood cholesterol level over these levels, there is an associated 2-3% rise in risk of stroke, heart attack, or sudden death. Men with cholesterol over 240 are at least three times more likely to have a heart attack than those whose cholesterol is under 160.

"...risk factors ...higher correlation to the LDL component..."

However, risk factors tend to have higher correlation to the LDL component of blood cholesterol than to the total cholesterol value. A LDL level below 160 mg/dL is advised if you have no major risk factors (such as low HDL levels, obesity, diabetes, smoking, or high blood pressure). If you do have major risk factors present, a LDL level below 140 mg/dL is recommended. Since having a normal cholesterol level is advantageous for most people, the following are some tips to help reduce blood cholesterol.

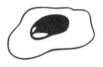

- Limit dietary cholesterol intake to no more than 300 mg per day. Avoid high cholesterol foods such as shellfish, liver and other organ meats. Reduce use of egg yolks and substitute egg whites or alternatives.
- Reduce saturated fats by reducing products of animal origin (such as fatty meats and high-fat dairy products). Use modest amounts of polyunsaturated oils and margarines as part of an overall lowfat diet.
- Have your cholesterol level checked by your doctor.
- Maintain a healthy weight. If overweight, talk with your physician about losing weight.
- Plan meals carefully to avoid high-fat foods, looking for lower fat alternatives and ways of cooking. Read food labels. Watch for ingredients on the higher saturated fat list. Trim fat from poultry and meats.

TABLE 14

"Exercise... can help lower cholesterol."

High Cholesterol Foods to Avoid			
Whole Milk Dairy Products	butter	cream (sweet or sour)	cream cheese
	custard	eggnog	high-fat cheese (American, cheddar)
	ice cream	whole milk	pudding
Animal Fat Sources	bacon	cold cuts	eggs (3 per week)
	fast foods	fried foods	gravies
	lard	marbled beef, lamb, pork	organ meats
	sauces	sausage	shellfish
Other Saturated Fats	coconut oil	palm oil	hydrogenated (hardened) fat

- Make your own dressings, desserts and sauces using ingredients which are lower in saturated fats. Such items purchased in stores and restaurants are usually high in fat and cholesterol.
- Eat more fresh fruit, whole grain breads and cereals, and vegetables. Regularly substitute vegetarian dishes for meat ones.
- Exercise (if sustained, vigorous, and regular) can help lower cholesterol.

Oils

If you must use an oil, make your selection carefully. Saturated fats are usually solid at room temperature and are usually found in animal products, but they also can be found in certain vegetable oils, including coconut oil and hydrogenated palm oil products. Polyunsaturated fats, liquid at room temperature, come from vegetable sources. Mono-unsaturated oils include canola oil and oils from olives, avocados, and peanuts and are believed to be beneficial in lowering heart disease risk, particularly if they replace a lot of saturated fat in our dietary intake.

"...oils should be used in moderation."

No matter whether mono- or polyunsaturated, oils should be used in moderation. Reasonable choices could include canola oil, and cottonseed, corn, olive, safflower, sunflower, and partially hydrogenated soybean oils. Be a label reader and select fat-reduced polyunsaturated or canola margarines, especially those where liquid oil is the first ingredient listed. Reduce the quantity of margarine used and try to avoid butter and stick margarine.

Notice in **graph 1** below that *coconut oil* (found in many products) has over *twice* the amount of *saturated fat* as does *lard*! You may also find other surprising comparisons. The chart lists oils in decreasing percentage of *saturated* fat.

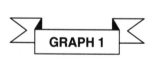

GRAPH 1

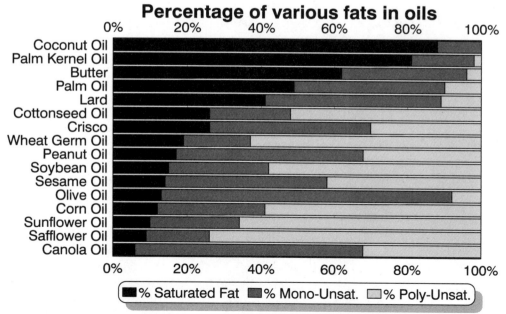

Percentage of various fats in oils

Vitamins & Minerals

Vitamins

Vitamins are organic compounds that are required in trace amounts in order to sustain good health. The National Institutes of Health set forth the well known *Recommended Daily Allowances* of vitamins, which are the amounts felt necessary to prevent disease (deficiency) states.

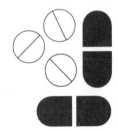

It is advisable to take a multivitamin and mineral supplement daily *if on caloric reduction* when attempting to lose weight. This is especially true if on low- or very- low calorie diets based on regular foods rather than on specially formulated or fortified products and if you feel tired and irritable. Iron and calcium supplementation needs special attention in women. [Keeping a food diary should also help you to monitor nutrient intake to assess adequate protein, carbohydrate, and fat intake during this process.]

> **FICTION**: If you take a vitamin and mineral supplement daily, a balanced diet is not a necessity.
> **FACT**: A balanced dietary intake of protein, carbohydrate, and fat is *always* essential for health. Such balanced intake usually provides nutritional amounts of needed vitamins and minerals, particularly on a maintenance program.

Just because an item starts out in its natural state with vitamins and minerals, does not mean it will keep its nutritive value if prepared or stored *improperly* or for too long. To acquire and preserve vitamins and nutrients, try the following:

"Do not overcook vegetables."

- Avoid prolonged soaking of fresh vegetables.
- Do not overcook vegetables. Try steaming or pressure-cooking them, rather than boiling or frying.
- Prepare salads just before you eat them.
- Use fresh fruits and vegetables over frozen or canned ones.
- Eat whole-grain cereals and bread versus refined ones.
- Consume brown rice instead of the white variety.
- Realize potatoes lose some of their nutritive value the longer they sit around.
- Store perishable items in your refrigerator (or freezer when appropriate). This might include seeds, nuts, produce, bread, flour, and oils in sealed containers.

The following are some selected vitamins and a very brief listing of some of their functions and benefits:

Vitamin A (retinol) — found in foods of animal origin. Yellow pigmented vegetables contain *carotene* (though vegetable itself may not be yellow—such as dark green leafy ones) which is converted to vitamin A in the body. Suppresses chemically induced tumors and functions in vision (dim light), growth, reproduction, membrane stability, cell differentiation, and maturation.

Vitamin B_1 (thiamine) — found in foods both of animal and vegetable origin. It is important in carbohydrate metabolism, digestion, growth, learning capacity, and muscle tone maintenance.

Vitamin B_2 (riboflavin) — found in legumes, brewer's yeast, nuts, whole grains, and other sources. Important for antibody and red blood cell formation, iron usage, and metabolic functions.

Vitamin B_3 (niacin) — cofactor for many enzymes and important in glycogen breakdown, tissue respiration, and sex hormone production. Large doses have been found to lower serum cholesterol but may have other *side-effects*. Deficiency of niacin leads to pellagra.

Vitamin B_6 (pyridoxine) — found in foods both of animal and vegetable origin. It is a cofactor for many enzymes and is involved in the metabolism of amino acids. It also plays a role in antibody formation, DNA & RNA synthesis, fat and protein utilization, and hemoglobin production.

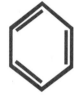

Vitamin C (ascorbic acid) — necessary for collagen formation (a supporting protein), wound healing, and important in several enzyme reactions. May lower risk of cancer of the stomach and esophagus and also increase iron absorption from food.

Vitamin D (calciferol) — promotes the absorption of calcium from the gut and is important to maintain proper calcium and phosphorus balance. Deficiency leads to rickets. This vitamin is important for normal bone growth and maintenance, blood clotting and proper function of the nervous system.

Vitamin E (tocopherol) — prevalent in vegetable oils, fresh greens, and other vegetables. Helps form red blood cells, muscle and other tissue. Essential for integrity of membranes and considered an antioxidant. One study showed the least carotid artery wall thickening with this vitamin. Other studies have suggested protection from certain forms of cancer.

Sodium

"We need as little as... 1/10 teaspoon salt..."

Sodium, an essential element for life, is found in greatest bodily concentrations in fluids outside of our individual cells. There it functions in one of its primary roles as being an osmotic (fluid-controlling) agent to maintain equilibrium between fluids inside our cells and fluids outside our cells. It is also important in our nerves and muscles working properly, along with some assistance from potassium and magnesium.

This mineral accounts for about 40% of the weight of salt and is measured in milligrams (mg). For example: 1 gram (1000 mg) salt = 400 mg sodium. One teaspoon of salt has 6 grams (2400 mg sodium). We need as little as 220 mg of sodium daily under normal circumstances, which is the amount in 1/10 teaspoon salt, or 2 slices of bread, or 3/4 cup cornflakes, or 2 cups of milk.

We acquire this necessary mineral through foods of animal and plant origin. As Americans, we acquire much of our sodium through table salt (either during cooking or before eating), certain products and processing chemicals, and even our water supply (concentration depends on our locality).

Sodium, like sugar, can be listed by many names. Ones to watch for on labels include baking powder, baking soda, brine, garlic salt, kelp, monosodium glutamate (MSG), sea salt, sodium chloride (table salt), sodium citrate, sodium nitrate, sodium phosphate, sodium saccharin, and soy sauce.

There is enough sodium present in naturally-occurring foods to meet our needs without adding extra salt. However, those engaged in strenuous work or exercise (especially in hot conditions), may lose sodium through heavy perspiration and need extra quantities. It is important to be aware of the fact that there are over 70 sodium compounds being used in foods today. It is found in antacids (sodium bicarbonate), baking soda/powder, beverages, butter, cheese, condiments, milk, monosodium glutamate (MSG), pickled foods, processed foods, sandwich meats, sauces, and snacks.

"...2/3 of our sodium intake is hidden..."

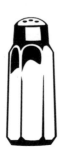

Possibly as much as 2/3 of our sodium intake is *hidden* in the processed foods we consume, with the other 1/3 coming from the salt shaker. Be aware of hidden sodium as many processed foods high in sodium may not taste salty. For example, one slice of brand-name white bread (123 mg) has as much sodium as 13 potato chips (124 mg). A chocolate McDonald's milk shake has more sodium (240 mg) than a medium serving of French fries (150 mg). One ounce of dry roasted mixed nuts has 190 mg sodium, but one cup of tomato soup has 932 mg sodium. Many water supplies have low sodium (under 5 mg/cup) but drier areas like Southern California can go as high as 20 mg/cup. Sodium in soft drinks and bottled waters range from 2-50 mg per cup. Remember that water softeners add sodium to the water.

Food sources **HIGH** in sodium:

- antacids containing sodium bicarbonate (e.g. Alka-Seltzer)
- bouillon cubes
- bread
- butter
- canned fish
- canned juice—tomato and V-8 vegetable juice
- canned vegetables/salads/beans
- cheese
- condiments
- deli salads with dressing
- frozen or packaged meals
- margarine
- meats—bacon, ham, luncheon meats, hot dogs, smoked meats
- olives
- pickles
- salad dressings
- sauces
- sauerkraut
- seasoning salts—celery, garlic, etc.
- snack foods—corn and potato chips, pretzels
- soups—canned or dry

Foods **MODERATE** in Sodium:

- breakfast cereals (<200 mg/serving)
- chocolate candy
- eggs
- fish, meat, or poultry that haven't been processed
- fruit and nut bars
- milk
- peanut butter
- *reduced sodium* products
- yogurt

Foods **LOW** in Sodium:

- alcohol
- beans & lentils—dried
- candy—hard
- chewing gum
- coffee
- corn and popcorn—unsalted
- fruit juices
- fruits and vegetables—fresh
- fruits—canned and dried
- herbs
- honey
- jam
- *low sodium* labeled products
- nuts and seeds—unsalted
- pasta—plain
- pepper
- potatoes
- rice
- *sodium-free* labeled products
- spices
- syrup
- tea
- tofu
- water

For adults with normal blood pressure, the American Heart Association recommends 1 gram (1000 mg) of sodium per 1000 calorie daily intake, not to exceed 3 grams a day. This is the amount you would get in one and one-fourth teaspoons of salt. The average American consumes 4000-6000 mg sodium per day (2-3 teaspoons of salt). Try to wean yourself off gradually, which will allow your taste buds to become more sensitive and actually allow you to notice the natural sodium and good taste of foods.

"Try to wean yourself off gradually..."

Excess sodium in the diet is associated with extra risk of developing high blood pressure, which in turn greatly increases risk of kidney failure, congestive heart failure, coronary heart disease, and stroke. Our kidneys normally get rid of excess dietary sodium, but *salt-sensitive* persons (possibly 1/3 of adults) tend to hold on to excess sodium (> 3000 mg/day) instead of excreting it. These are the ones at greater risk for hypertension. Those with normal blood pressure and no risk factors for elevated blood pressure (such as diabetes, obesity, being black, or family history) may not have an urgent need to limit salt, but moderation between 2-4 grams daily intake is a good goal.

Check labels for sodium levels. Most canned soups have 800 to 1,000 mg. of sodium per serving. The following terms may appear on products:
   Reduced Sodium: at least 75% less sodium than the original product.
   Low Sodium: 140 mg or less per serving.
   Very Low Sodium: 35 mg or less per serving.
   Sodium Free: Less than 5 mg per serving.

"Learn to enjoy the natural flavor..."

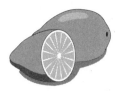

Tips to reduce sodium levels in our dietary intake:

- Avoid antacids with sodium bicarbonate (e.g. Alka-Seltzer) as they are high in sodium. Don't swallow mouth washes or toothpaste as most contain sodium.
- Watch the table salt. You can limit sodium there by 50% if you substitute something like Morton's Lite Salt, or try something like a sodium-free herb-spice blend (e.g. Mrs. Dash). NOTE: Potassium salt substitutes may not be suitable for some persons—check with your doctor.
- Go easy on sauces and condiments like soy sauce, salad dressings, spaghetti sauces, ketchup, bottled peppers, and mustard. Hunt for the low sodium varieties.
- Rinse canned vegetables and beans before using them to remove excess salt.
- Do not salt your children's food to your taste.
- Learn to enjoy the natural flavor of unsalted food. Taste your food before salting it.
- Use lemon/citrus juice or herbs and spices to flavor foods. Dry mustard, nutritional yeast, garlic, peppers, onions, or even a little cooking wine all add extra flavor without the sodium. Cook without salt or just use a small amount (1/2 the recipe amount). Try garlic, celery, or onion *power* instead of the *salt* variety.
- Limit: bacon, bouillon (regular), cheese, cured meats, diet sodas, ham, hot dogs, luncheon meats, olives, pickled foods, processed foods (potato chips, pretzels, salted nuts, canned soups and vegetables, etc.), sausage, soy sauce, steak sauce, and commercial tomato sauce.
- Substitute low sodium products for higher sodium ones. Use sodium reduced breads, butter, and margarine. Regular varieties may contain up to 2% salt.
- Choose plain popcorn, fresh or dried fruits, and unsalted nuts or seeds.
- When dining out, request dishes without added salt. Remember most fast-food items are high in sodium content.

Calcium

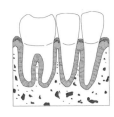

Calcium is a mineral necessary for healthy bones and teeth (which store 99% of our body's calcium). It also plays a vital role in muscle and nerve function, blood clotting, insulin secretion, enzyme regulation, and overall bone strength. It may even help to lower blood pressure. Studies show those with < 300 mg calcium per day have a 2-3 times increased risk of developing hypertension compared to those with 1200 mg intake.

Many foods contain calcium, such as green leafy vegetables (cabbage, broccoli), dried beans, legumes, nuts, tofu (soybean curd), whole-grain cereal, canned fish with edible bones (tuna, sardines, salmon), milk, yogurt, and cheese. Be sure to select lowfat dairy products, such as lowfat cottage cheese, non-fat yogurt, or skim milk. These are low in saturated fat and contain as much calcium as whole milk.

Those who have trouble eating enough calcium-rich foods should consider a calcium supplement, usually taken with a meal. People with a history of *kidney stones* should talk to their doctor before significantly increasing calcium intake.

There are some factors you should be aware of that might lead to *poor calcium* absorption or retention by the body. These include:

- exercise deficiency
- fat excess
- menopausal hormone changes
- protein excess
- salt excess
- smoking
- vitamin-D deficiency

Current dietary calcium recommendations for persons over 19 years of age are 800 mg per day. Men over 50 should take 1000 mg per day. Some authorities believe that women should consume 1,000 to 1,500 milligrams daily, well before the menopause. These same authorities feel that postmenopausal women should consume 1,000 mg. of calcium daily if they are receiving estrogen therapy, and 1,500 mg. daily if they are not. Taking excess calcium really is of no benefit once the body's calcium needs are met. For example, bones are not made any stronger. In fact, excessive amounts (> 3000 mg/day) can interfere with iron absorption.

Osteoporosis - Calcium relationship

Osteoporosis is derived from a Latin term. It is a condition whereby bones become thin, brittle, and fragile and can fracture easily. It occurs almost eight times more frequently in women as in men. Bone density usually builds until we reach our thirties, after which there begins a gradual loss of bone mass. The stronger our bones are as this loss begins, the fewer problems that should occur later. In most cases, there often are no symptoms of bone loss and 30-40 years may go by before the first bone fracture occurs. It is known that the chief risk factor is age and the earlier treatment or prevention of this process occurs, the greater the benefit.

Blood calcium level is usually kept constant by the steady interchange of this mineral between bone and blood. When there is inadequate calcium obtained from our diet, the body drains calcium out of the bones. This calcium loss from the bones over the years may lead to osteoporosis, literally *porous bones*, a condition of thinning and structural weakening of the bones.

TABLE 15

Good Sources of Calcium		
Item	Amount	Milligrams
Yogurt	8 oz.	415
Sardines	4 oz.	400
Ricotta cheese	1/2 cup	335
Milk	8 oz.	270
Cheese (cheddar)	1 oz.	204
Greens, collard	1/2 cup	178
Broccoli	1 cup	177
Greens, turnip	1/2 cup	133
Tofu	4 oz.	102
Dried beans	1 cup (cooked)	90

"Bone density ...builds until we reach our thirties..."

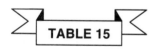

The affected bones tend to become weak, frail, and easy to fracture. This is especially true regarding the spinal vertebrae, hip, and wrist bones. Loss of body height and development of spine curvature may result, as can periodontal disease with resulting jaw bone deterioration affecting support of the teeth. Today, *more women die* from the effects and complications of osteoporosis than from cancer of the breast and cervix combined.

Females seem to be especially susceptible to osteoporosis, which affects 1 in 4 by age 65 causing loss of *over half* their bone density. Women have about 30% less bone than men and lose bone at a faster rate after menopause due to decreased estrogen hormone. By the time a woman reaches her eighties, she may have lost up to two-thirds of her skeleton.

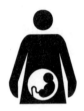

Pregnancy and breast-feeding place *additional calcium demands* on the woman that must be met. Otherwise, osteoporosis will become an even greater risk due to calcium bone reserves being utilized more than normal. Other items contributing to osteoporosis may include some or all of the following factors:

- caffeine
- Caucasian women who are small-boned and light-skinned (genetics)
- certain anticonvulsant medications
- consumption of soft drinks, junk food, and excess salt (nutritional factors)
- excess alcohol
- excess phosphorus (from meat & soft drinks)
- gender
- insufficient calcium in the diet
- insufficient vitamin-D
- lack of weight-bearing exercise (physical activity)
- ovaries removed or non-functioning (menopause)
- prolonged use of aluminum containing antacids
- sex hormones (estrogen, testosterone)
- smoking
- thin women tend to have higher osteoporosis risk than obese women

"...do things that build strong, dense bones."

One key to prevention is to do things that build strong, dense bones. Young women may be able to reduce this risk by consuming high-calcium foods and/or supplements, and utilizing regular weight-bearing exercise. Hormone therapy for post-menopausal women may be prescribed by some physicians to help delay osteoporosis.

In most published studies about calcium, the relationship between bone density and dietary calcium consumption has been weak or nonexistent. However, many health professionals feel that even if dietary calcium cannot reverse age-related bone loss, it may help to slow the process.

"...Americans are heavily into dietary protein..."

Since calcium and osteoporosis are intertwined, and since Americans are heavily into dietary protein and fats, it is significant that some research, medical editorials, and journals are warning of protein intake causing a negative calcium balance (increases loss of calcium). They are reporting that no matter how much calcium we take in, the more protein in our dietary intake—the more calcium we lose. One long-term project found that with as little as 75 grams of daily protein, more calcium is lost in the urine than is absorbed by the body through dietary intake.

Countries where large amounts of calcium and dairy products are consumed have much higher rates of osteoporosis than countries where little calcium and little or no dairy products are consumed. In America, those eating 20 percent of their calories from protein may be assuring themselves a negative mineral balance (loss), not just in calcium, but also in iron, zinc, and magnesium. It may be directly affected by how much protein is consumed.

Chromium

Chromium is a mineral that is important for normal glucose metabolism. It may be useful for appetite control, particularly *sweet cravings* (sugars and carbohydrates). Some have suggested that it may be important for *fat burning hormones* and preventing fat rebound after weight loss. Gary Evans (a former USDA researcher) feels chromium picolinate decreases body fat and increases lean muscle mass [personal communication].

"Chromium ...important for normal glucose metabolism."

Chromium *picolinate* is one of the best absorbed forms that can be taken as a supplement. Somes sources have recommended a dose of one to three of the 200 mcg. pills daily. Chromium *polynicotinate* is not absorbed as well as the picolinate version according to Mr. Evans. Dietary sources of chromium include animal foods, whole-grain products, and certain types of yeast.

Potassium

Potassium is an essential electrolyte needed by the body for many functions. Daily needs are about 2,000 mg for adults. It is found in its highest concentrations within the cells (in contrast to sodium). There has been evidence that in some patients, increasing dietary potassium may lower blood pressure and reduce the hypertensive effect of excess sodium.

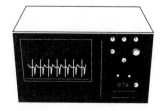

During weight loss utilizing low-calorie or very-low-calorie diets, this is one of the primary electrolytes that tends to become depleted. Depletion is also increased with vomiting, diarrhea, and similar problems. Sources of dietary potassium include dried apricots, avocados, baby lima beans, bananas, broccoli, carrots, dates, figs, juices (orange, prune, tomato), potatoes, raisins, spinach, and *lite salt* substitutes.

Iron

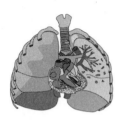

Iron is a very important mineral whose main function is to carry oxygen from the lungs to the tissues of the body. Sources of iron include a wide variety of plant and animal foods. In red blood cells, iron combines with protein to form hemoglobin—the oxygen carrying red pigment. About two-thirds of our body's iron is utilized for this production of hemoglobin. The remainder is found in enzymes, muscles, and other tissues.

Iron deficiency is one of the most prevalent nutritional deficiencies in women. Those between 11 and 50 years of age are at greater risk of this deficiency due to the monthly loss of menstrual blood. Growth, endurance sports, and pregnancy also increase the body's requirements for iron. The risk of iron deficiency is also increased in dieters who don't eat well-balanced meals. Therefore, these categories of people may benefit from an iron supplement. Consult your physician.

"Iron deficiency ...prevalent ...in women."

Chronic shortage of this mineral can limit production of hemoglobin and hence the amount of oxygen carried to the body cells (can be part of anemia). Oxygen-starved tissues in anemia can produce the following symptoms:

- skin paleness
- breathlessness
- attention span decrease

- fatigue or excessive tiredness
- malaise and irritability
- always feeling cold

Excessive iron intake (above 70 mg per day) can be toxic, so be aware of recommended daily amounts, as shown in the chart. Iron absorption is *enhanced by* vitamin C-containing fruits, vegetables, and salads eaten with the meal. Small amounts of poultry, fish, or meat help to absorb iron from vegetables. Absorption is *reduced by* excessive bran fiber, calcium supplements, and tea (tannin) consumed within one hour of a meal.

TABLE 16

Recommended Daily Iron Intake	
Age	**Iron**
Males: 11-18 y.o.	12 mg
19+	10 mg
Females: 11-50 y.o.	15 mg
51+	10 mg

"Excessive iron intake can be toxic..."

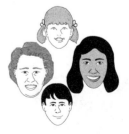

Beverages

Fluid

Possibly one of the most neglected, least understood, and fairly important guidelines involved in weight reduction is that of water intake and fluid balance. Our bodies are about *seventy percent water*. An average person consumes three times their body weight in water every seven months. Water comes from water consumption, beverages, and solid foods. The body also manufactures water during metabolism.

We are all aware of the importance of water and proper fluid intake, yet so many Americans neglect this important area. It becomes even more important for those attempting to reduce weight. Water helps to suppress the appetite naturally and helps the body to metabolize stored fat. Many times we misinterpret *thirst* as hunger. Next time you feel like snacking, try sipping on a glass of water instead.

Research has shown that a *decrease* in fluid intake will cause fat deposits to *increase*, while increasing fluid intake can cause a *reduction* in fat stores. One explanation for this phenomenon is that our kidneys need plenty of fluid to function properly. When they don't work to capacity (inadequate fluid), some of their work is sent to the liver. Since one function of the liver is to metabolize stored fat into usable energy for the rest of the body, taking on additional work from the kidney won't allow it to metabolize fat at peak efficiency. As a result, less fat is metabolized, more fat remains stored, and weight loss slows or stops.

Besides helping the kidney to operate more efficiently, the body uses fluid (water) for other uses, such as:

"You need a minimum of 64 oz. of fluid daily."

- carry vital substances to cells
- carry wastes away from cells (very important in fat breakdown)
- ensure proper functioning of digestive juices and digestive tract
- help to prevent skin sagging that usually accompanies weight loss
- lubricate joint surfaces and internal organs
- maintenance of proper muscle tone
- moisten lungs and respiratory tract
- regulate body temperature (if very hot, may lose one quart of water per hour)

You need a minimum of 64 oz of fluid daily (8-10 glasses). Some advocate at least 10 to 12 eight ounce glasses of water per day, plus one extra glass for every 25 pounds over your ideal weight. Water is suggested since it tends to be the lowest in sodium and calories (0) compared to other drinks. Other beverages can be used, but count their calories. Don't underestimate the importance of this fluid intake and don't forget that certain disease processes, such as diarrhea, vomiting, hyperventilation, and high fevers can cause a loss of up to several quarts of water a day.

If this sounds like a lot of water, especially if you only drink one glass a day, take heart. You don't have to jump to ten glasses overnight. Start with an assessment of

"Drink two glasses of fluid at each meal."

how much fluids you currently consume (fluid diary). Then, add an extra glass to your current amount every two or three days. After a certain amount, you will reach a *breakthrough point* when you will notice a craving for fluids, you may drop several pounds as your body starts a natural diuresis, and you might notice less fluid retention (if this has been a problem in the past). Obviously, if you have a medical condition (e.g. kidney or heart failure) requiring fluid restriction, check with your physician before increasing fluid intake.

Other water consumption tips include:

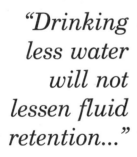

- Drink a large glass of water prior to each meal, perhaps 20 minutes or so, to help fill your stomach and help slow down overeating.
- Drink two glasses of fluid at each meal. This will assure at least six glasses of fluid daily. Adding just two or three more glasses throughout the day will then get you to the recommended amount of fluid intake.
- Avoid alcohol when reducing weight. Avoid regular soft drinks and limit fruit juice (1 glass has the calories of 2-3 pieces of fresh fruit). Use diet drinks in moderation, especially those containing caffeine.
- When considering fluids, you can use some low-calorie, no caffeine beverage such as Crystal Light or mineral water. Remember decaffeinated doesn't mean caffeine-free—just less caffeine than the regular beverage.

Lowfat buttermilk, skim milk, or plain lowfat yogurt can provide an excellent base for a nutritious beverage. Blend these dairy products with fresh or unsweetened frozen fruits and a little sweetener, if needed. If you wish a texture closer to a milkshake, add cracked ice and blend.

"Drinking less water will not lessen fluid retention..."

Water balance in our bodies is controlled by water (fluid) intake and output, amount of sodium ingested, and *Aldosterone* (a hormone). If water intake is inadequate, the body will secrete aldosterone to conserve as much sodium and water as it can. When people consume more than the recommended 3000 mg sodium a day, they tend to retain the extra sodium, along with associated fluid retention. Certain medications (e.g. anti-inflammatory) and obesity can also promote this tendency to fluid retention. Inadequate intake makes the body function as if it were in a drought, holding on to every drop and storing it in tissue spaces outside of the cells. This becomes apparent as swelling in the hands, feet, and legs.

With this sort of fluid retention, diuretics (fluid pills) become only a temporary solution. They force out stored water along with some nutrients. Again, this appears as a threat to the body and it replaces lost water at the first opportunity, causing the fluid retention to return.

Therefore, if a person has normal kidney and heart function, drinking extra water becomes a good treatment for fluid retention as it allows the body to rid itself of extra fluid. Drinking less water *will not lessen* fluid retention; it only aggravates it.

Caffeine

Caffeine is a plant alkaloid that occurs naturally in some plants. It is quickly absorbed by the body and reaches peak levels within 30 to 60 minutes after ingestion. While most people are aware that caffeine is found in coffee beans, cola nuts, tea, and cocoa beans, some may find it surprising that it can also be found in many over-the-counter and prescription medications, as well as chocolate and many carbonated drinks (not just colas).

It can cause an increase in appetite, blood pressure (especially during exercise), urine output, respiration rate, digestive secretions, heart rate, and worsen symptoms of fibrocystic breast disease. It can also affect the central nervous system by increasing anxiety and restlessness and by delaying fatigue. Caffeine can cause an overstimulation of the adrenal glands. Those who consume high levels of caffeine may develop a *withdrawal syndrome* if it is stopped abruptly. Some of the negative side effects that could be experienced include: depression, diarrhea, headache, hyperactivity, insomnia, and irritability.

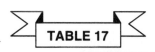

TABLE 17

Caffeine Content of Various Drinks

ITEM	CAFFEINE (mg)
Coffee (5 oz. cup)	
Drip method	137-153
Percolated	97-125
Instant, Freeze Dried	61-70
Decaffeinated	1-9
Tea (5 oz. cup)	
One-minute brew	9-33
Three-minute brew	20-46
Five-minute brew	24-55
Herbal tea	0
Coca (1 oz.)	
Milk chocolate	15
Baking chocolate, unsweetened	25
Soft Drinks (12 oz.)	
Coca-Cola	61
Dr. Pepper	58
Mello Yello	52
Mountain Dew	51
Diet Coke	46
TAB	44
Pepsi Cola	41
Diet Pepsi	34
RC Cola	31
Diet Rite	0

Caffeine Levels in Drug Preparations

ITEM	Caffeine (mg. per tablet)*
Over-the-counter Stimulants	
No Doz	100
Vivarin	200
Pain Relievers	
Advil	0
Anacin	32
Excedrin Extra-strength	65
Midol original	32
Vanquish	33
Aspirin, plain	0
Prescription Pain Relievers	
Cafergot	100
Darvon Compound	32.4
Feldene	0
Fiorinal	40

*Information from PDR & PDR for Nonprescription Drugs

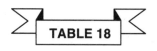

TABLE 18

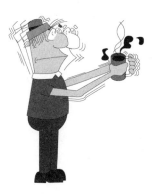

Alcohol

If you are maintaining weight and drink alcoholic beverages, do so in moderation because they are high in calories and low in nutrients. If attempting to reduce weight, any excess of these *non-nutrient* calories wastes some of your daily calorie allotment and contributes nothing to satisfy true hunger. Don't be fooled into thinking wine coolers will help reduce weight as the typical 12 oz. bottle has more alcohol than either a 12 oz. can of beer, a 5 oz. glass of wine, or an ounce of liquor. Alcohol has also been known to increase appetite, especially if consumed before a meal.

"Alcohol can also increase appetite..."

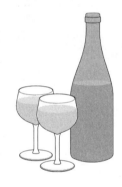

It is wise to *avoid all alcohol* during a weight reduction program as many patients find that even small amounts tend to markedly slow their ability to lose weight. It diverts dietary fat away from being burned and redirects it towards storage. Alcoholic drinks are *potentially more harmful* while on a low-calorie weight reduction program. Not consuming alcohol with medication is also a wise rule of thumb. Mental faculties and normal skills (such as driving) are more readily impaired. Alcohol can also *weaken your resolve* to eat properly.

Alcohol does raise good (HDL) cholesterol levels, which helps protect against arterial plaques and coronary artery disease. However, having more than one or two alcoholic drinks daily was associated with minimal reduction of risk of coronary artery disease and it actually increased other risks such as strokes, heart and liver problems, and high blood pressure. Women with higher alcohol consumption tend to have more abdominal (central; android) fat, along with increased health risks. Alcohol influences the association between central (abdominal) fat distribution and plasma androgens in premenopausal women and can also lead to higher risks of certain women's breast disease.

The American Heart Association recommends alcohol drinkers consume less than 1 and 1/2 oz of pure alcohol daily. This is equivalent to 3 oz of 100-proof whiskey, two 12 oz beers, or two 4 oz glasses of wine.

As mentioned earlier, you should also watch *calories* from alcohol. The higher the proof, the higher the alcohol content (and calorie content). Some bottled wine coolers may contain 150 to 300 calories. Mix drinks with club soda or diet ginger ale to help reduce calories. Refilling your glass with more soda when half empty will keep down the calorie count and make it last longer.

> **FICTION:** Alcoholic beverages don't contribute to weight. After all, you rarely see a fat alcoholic.
> **FACT:** Alcohol is high in non-nutritional calories and can cause weight gain. It often is an appetite stimulant, which contributes to eating even more calories. Alcoholics generally neglect other nutritional needs to consume alcohol, thereby losing weight through very unhealthy and inappropriate means.

Free Foods

For the most part, *free foods* are food items that have the *lowest calories* and are *good filler foods*. Consider snacking on them when you have the urge to sample meals you are preparing. These foods can be eaten *as desired* to add more variety to any dietary management program. While the listings in the table below are not *all* of the foods considered to be part of this category, they should get you started thinking along the right track. Just seek out less calorie dense foods and you will be on your way to successful weight management.

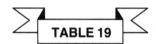

TABLE 19

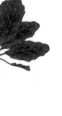
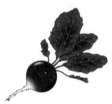
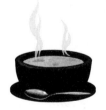
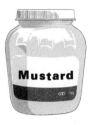

Vegetables (1/2 cup)	Asparagus (6 spears)	Beet greens	Broccoli
	Cabbage	Cauliflower	Celery
	Chard	Cucumber	Dandelion greens
	Endive	Escarole	Lettuce
	Parsley	Peppers	Pickles--sour, dill & unsweetened
	Pimentos	Radishes	Rhubarb
	Sauerkraut	Spinach	Squash, summer
	Turnip greens	Watercress	
Beverages	Coffee, black, no sugar	Tea, plain, no sugar	Carbonated water
	Mineral water	Non-calorie, flavored drink	
Soups	Bouillon	Clear soups without fat	Consommé
Sweeteners	Sugar substitutes	Saccharin	Sucaryl
Relishes	Bread & butter pickles	Cucumber pickles	Dill pickles
	India relish	Pickled onions	Sour pickles
Seasonings	Celery salt	Chives	Dill
	Monosodium glutamate	Horse-radish	Lemon, juice, sections or slices
	Mustard	Pepper	Salt (use sparingly)
	Sauces, like Worcestershire	Tobasco	Spices
	Vinegar	Garlic	

Pyramid Guide

In April, 1992, the Department of Agriculture finally unveiled its new *Food Guide Pyramid*, after being delayed for awhile. A pyramid structure was chosen because it gave more space and emphasis to the *foundational* bread, grain, and cereal group than to the *supplemental* dairy, meat, and high-protein group. It was designed to replace the traditional *Basic Four Food Groups* charts that tended to give *equal emphasis* to meat, milk, grains, and fruits and vegetables.

The guide follows the recommendations of the Dietary Guidelines for Americans: wide food variety; consume less salt, sugar, and fat; eat more fresh fruit and vegetables, wholegrain breads and cereals; and drink less alcohol. It should be emphasized that *Americans talk lean but eat fat*! We should do what we can to learn more healthful eating styles and then practice what we've learned. For example, only 9% of American adults eat five fruit and vegetable servings a day, the amount recommended by the pyramid.

"...we don't need to consume as much protein..."

The large base shows that the largest dietary consumption should be from breads, cereals, rice, pasta, and other starchy foods, suggesting 6 to 11 servings from this category. The groups next in importance in supporting good health are the vegetables and fruits, with 3 to 5 daily servings of vegetables and 2 to 4 servings of fruits suggested.

The design then tapers to help us visualize that we don't need to consume as much protein as we currently do. It suggests 2 to 3 daily servings of milk and dairy products and meat, poultry, fish, and other protein foods (beans, eggs, nuts, seeds) and places these groups near the top of the pyramid.

At the very top of the pyramid, the last group is labeled *use sparingly* and consists of fats, oils, and sweets. In other words, consume these in *very small amounts* to liven up other foods or only on *less frequent* occasions.

How to Use The Daily Food Guide

What counts as one serving?

Breads, Cereals, Rice, and Pasta
1 slice of bread
1/2 cup of cooked rice or pasta
1/2 cup of cooked cereal
1 ounce of ready-to-eat cereal

Vegetables
1/2 cup of chopped raw or
  cooked vegetables
1 cup of leafy raw vegetables

Fruits
1 piece of fruit or melon wedge
3/4 cup of juice
1/2 cup of canned fruit
1/4 cup of dried fruit

Milk, Yogurt, and Cheese
1 cup of milk or yogurt
1-1/2 to 2 ounces of cheese

Meat, Poultry, Fish, Dry Beans, Eggs, and Nuts
2-1/2 to 3 ounces of cooked lean
  meat, poultry, or fish
Count 1/2 cup of cooked beans,
  or 1 egg, or 2 tablespoons of
  peanut butter as 1 ounce of lean
  meat (about 1/3 serving)

Fats, Oils, and Sweets
LIMIT CALORIES FROM THESE
especially if you need to lose weight

The amount you eat may be more than one serving. For example, a dinner portion of spaghetti would count as two or three servings of pasta.

Food Guide Pyramid

A Guide to Daily Food Choices

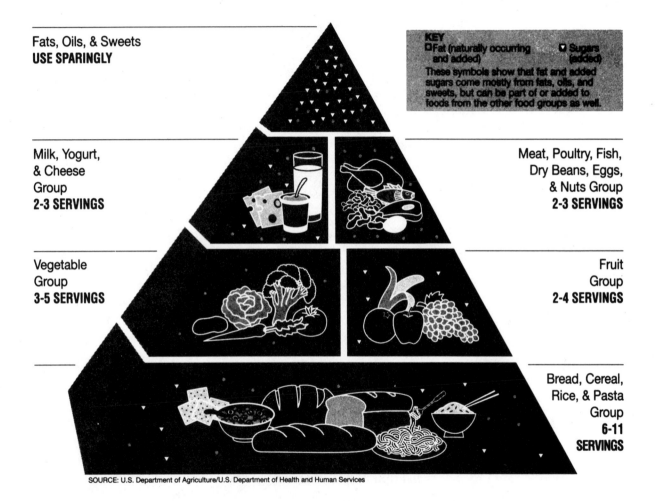

Fats, Oils, & Sweets
USE SPARINGLY

KEY
□ Fat (naturally occurring and added) ▽ Sugars (added)
These symbols show that fat and added sugars come mostly from fats, oils, and sweets, but can be part of or added to foods from the other food groups as well.

Milk, Yogurt, & Cheese Group
2-3 SERVINGS

Meat, Poultry, Fish, Dry Beans, Eggs, & Nuts Group
2-3 SERVINGS

Vegetable Group
3-5 SERVINGS

Fruit Group
2-4 SERVINGS

Bread, Cereal, Rice, & Pasta Group
6-11 SERVINGS

SOURCE: U.S. Department of Agriculture/U.S. Department of Health and Human Services

Use the Food Guide Pyramid to help you eat better every day. . .the Dietary Guidelines way. Start with plenty of Breads, Cereals, Rice, and Pasta; Vegetables; and Fruits. Add two to three servings from the Milk group and two to three servings from the Meat group.

Each of these food groups provides some, but not all, of the nutrients you need. No one food group is more important than another — for good health you need them all. Go easy on fats, oils, and sweets, the foods in the small tip of the Pyramid.

To order a copy of "The Food Guide Pyramid" booklet, send a $1.00 check or money order made out to the Superintendent of Documents to: Consumer Information Center, Department 159-Y, Pueblo, Colorado 81009.

U.S. Department of Agriculture, Human Nutrition Information Service, August 1992, Leaflet No. 572

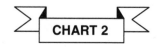

CHART 2

Eating

As you are modifying your behavior, lifestyle, and eating habits, realize that not every single thing you eat has to be healthy. There are no forbidden foods—only modifications in portions and frequency of some of them. Eating should be pleasurable, not guilt ridden and a source of constant frustration. Enjoy your foods and life, but do so in a healthy manner.

The following tips and suggestions are just that, suggestions. Some people need firm direction in order to modify behavior or eating so some phrases may be laced with *avoid, don't, try not to, omit* and other similar instructions. Take these in light of the statement in the paragraph above. Use them as guidelines, not the letter of the *food law*. Don't look at the structure set up by these tips, merely get into the spirit of them. Make small changes consistently rather than large changes inconsistently and you will succeed.

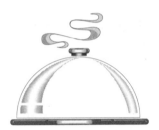

"Eating should be pleasurable..."

A general caloric rule-of-thumb is that the *smooth things take their toll* and the *crisp things help you reach your goal*. Putting it simply, smooth and creamy items— ice cream, pudding, butter, sour cream, bananas, gravy, oils, mayonnaise, mousses— tend to have higher calories (many times loaded with fats and hundreds of calories) that take their *toll* in excess weight and increased health risks. Crisp items—celery, cucumbers, dill pickles, lettuce, radishes, rice cakes— are lower in calories and can help you in your *goal* of weight management.

- Avoid:
    1) alcohol when dieting.
    2) fried foods, high-fat snacks and high-fat fast foods.
    3) regular soft drinks; use sugar-free diet drinks. Limit fruit juice.
    4) sugar and foods high in sugar such as fruit drinks, jams, chocolate, cookies, cakes, donuts, ice cream and ice-confections. Use artificial sweeteners and artificially sweetened diet products.
- Be mindful of *what* is going into your mouth, as well as *how often* your mouth has something in it.
- Don't:
    1) eat every bite of food on your plate. Leave something and show you are in control.
    2) eat leftovers on plates when cleaning up the kitchen. Put them in the garbage or store in opaque containers immediately.
    3) keep high fat foods in your house, car, or office.
- Drink as much water as possible.
- Eat:
    1) a variety of breads and cereals.
    2) a variety of foods, so you don't become bored.
    3) adequate fresh fruits, vegetables, and whole-grain cereal products.
    4) high-fat foods on a limited basis.
    5) more fruits, vegetables, and grains. They will help to fill you up.

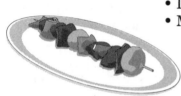

6) three moderate meals daily that are nutritionally balanced and avoid fad diets that continually come and go (just look at the multitude of these diets on magazines at the supermarket checkout stands). By spacing food intake throughout the day, you will let your body know that you are not depriving it of food, making it less likely to try to conserve by storing more fat.

- Get away from eating as a mindless, mechanical routine of shoveling food into your body. Slow down, reflect, and give thanks for food, life and a world full of opportunity.
- Have a positive attitude. You can do anything you really want to. You will never be happy with others unless you can be happy with yourself!
- If you are obsessed with food, get help. Call weight management groups or consult health specialists in your community.
- Limit nuts as they tend to be high in oils and fats.
- Make:
  1) problematic eating as difficult as possible. For example, prepare and eat only 1 slice of bread at a time. Put up the loaf and margarine each time.
  2) small changes. Don't try to change all your eating habits in one day or even one week.
- Modify everything you eat toward lower fat alternatives when possible.
- Omit regular butter and margarine from your diet.
- Plan for each meal rather than just grabbing haphazardly whatever looks good on the menu or in the refrigerator.
- Quench your thirst on water or mineral water.
- Read labels on everything before you buy or eat it.
- Remove:
  1) skin from poultry and trim fat from meat.
  2) your plate when you are finished so you aren't tempted to keep nibbling.
- Sit down when you eat. This will help you eat slower and take the time for your body and mind (satiety center) to experience eating satisfaction.
- Skipping meals may make you binge eat, snack more, or eat more at the meals you do eat.
- Some physiologists recommend that you should eat about every five hours to maintain a steady energy level. Hypoglycemics should have at least five equally-spaced meals instead of the traditional three daily.
- Take a multivitamin and mineral supplement daily if on low calories, particularly if irritable and tired.
- The earlier in the day you consume food (and calories), the better.
- There is no food that cannot occasionally be eaten; e.g. chocolate, cake, dessert, wine. It is the *amount* and *frequency* of eating it that is critical.
- Try:
  1) eating more slowly, enjoying your food and how it tastes.
  2) not to be so consumed with food. Try to think of it as fuel for your engine, instead of as a recreational sport.

"Have a positive attitude."

"Modify... toward lower fat..."

3) substituting more rice, potatoes, and pasta in place of high-fat meat and meat-products.
- Use:
    1) lowfat dairy products and low-calorie salad dressings.
    2) minimal amounts of fat and oil and utilize fat-free cooking whenever possible.
- When dining out, avoid fried and sauce-laden dishes as well as pastries, salad dressings and desserts. Eat moderately.

Preparation & Planning

The first step in preparation for healthier eating is to *remove all danger foods* from the home. Danger foods are those foods, snacks, or beverages over which you feel you have no willpower or control. If these remain in your house, it's only a matter of time before they find their way into your mouth (possibly during a binge). Either throw away or give away these foods.

"...remove all danger foods..."

If other members of your family need or demand these type of items, have them take and hide them from you. Better still, enlist their cooperation to help you by allowing you to keep them out of the house for six months or one year. Make it a contest with appropriate rewards for all involved.

Careful planning for meals ahead of time is the next step. People with weight problems need to be more mindful of what they are going to eat at mealtime and not make on-the-spot decisions. Try to buy only foods that require considerable preparation. Avoid the *quickie* snacks. Stick to a set menu (healthy game plan). Utilize beans, pasta, and rice as part of the main course, instead of just side dishes. You can prepare low-calorie *finger foods* ahead of time and keep them in clear, easy to open containers or zipper-bags in the front of the refrigerator. If some of these are cut up vegetables, you can use them for salads or just snacking at any time.

Have either a written or mental *list of non-food activities* that you can do if you become bored, depressed, tired, lonely, or frustrated. Simple things like reading, homecraft hobbies, taking a walk, single player sports, relaxation exercises, or calling a friend or neighbor are just a few suggestions.

Learn stress management techniques and how to really relax and deal with emotions and moods on a positive level (many hospitals and local organizations offer courses on this). Join a weight management group if you feel you need someone to share problems, frustrations, and exchange ideas with. Group support has been effective for many reducers.

Take low-calorie snacks, drinks, or food to the office or for parties. Learn to say "No, thank you" and feel good about yourself and your resolve. True friends will understand and appreciate your determination.

Shopping

Dietary shopping, like proper eating, sometimes requires *advance preparation*. One useful tool to help prepare for shopping is the shopping list. However, this list may be slightly different from your previous ones. The list I recommend has two columns, one for things *to buy* and the other column for things *not to buy*. In this very important second column, write down items you've been suckered by or overly tempted by. These things usually have little (if any) nutritional value, especially considering the price you spend for them.

EXAMPLE 3

By shopping with a list, this turns shopping into a disciplined activity, rather than a free-for-all. It should make shopping quicker, easier, and less expensive. You will then control shopping, instead of it controlling you through gimmicks and appeals to areas of vulnerability and weakness. Supermarkets are devised to create appeal and enticement to buy things whether you need them or not (see also a book entitled *The Hidden Persuaders*). Obviously you may depart from the list, but you should find yourself buying more nourishing foods and less junk ones.

"Supermarkets are devised to create appeal and enticement..."

Shopping List	
Buy More	**Buy Less**
chicken	butter
citrus & tomato juices	candy, cake, cookies
fish	commercial baked goods
fresh vegetables	fruit in heavy syrup
fruits	heavy marbled or processed meat
lowfat dairy products	
whole grain bread & rolls	ice cream
whole grain cereal	presweetened cereals
	snack foods

Surveys have shown that shopping from a list can limit in-store buying time to an average of 30 minutes. Those without a list averaged longer shopping times and higher bills. The amount spent in supermarkets averages about a dollar a minute. And remember, it's never too late to return something. Even if the cashier has rung up the sale, you can always change your mind and return an unneeded item. It's your health and your money.

While shopping habits for everyone can vary a little, there have been some general areas identified that tend to give most people trouble in keeping it nutritionally focused. Some of these are identified as follows, along with suggestions on how to counter them:

1) ***Shopping when hungry.*** Surveys confirm that hungry shoppers buy 20% more food (that they don't really need) than they would if not hungry. It also tends to be the wrong kind—already prepared, high calorie, and able to be eaten immediately.

   TIP: Don't shop when hungry. Eat a meal or healthy snack before you go. Even if not hungry, avoid aisles with packaged chips,

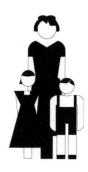

cookies, and sodas. If you don't see them, you won't be as tempted to purchase them.

2) *Shopping with children.* Kids may pressure you into buying things (snack, junk foods, etc.) that you ordinarily would not buy.
 TIP: Shop alone. Leave the kids at home or with a friend or neighbor. (Spouses may also make you buy more.)

3) *Buying the bargain giant economy size.* Many times in an effort to save money, you may actually over-buy items. You then feel guilty if it isn't all finished at a meal and may tend to consume the unneeded left-overs.
 TIP: Do unit pricing to see if the larger size is *really* a bargain. Many products may actually cost the same or more per unit (ounce, item, etc.). Purchasing larger quantities is only a bargain if you don't eat the extra helpings or have to throw out spoiled leftovers.

4) *Buying items with coupons that would not normally be purchased.* Manufacturers know that coupons may entice people to purchase their product, using pricing as a gimmick to bait you.
 TIP: Throw away coupons you don't really need and check newspaper specials before going shopping. Try to keep the *buy—don't buy* list in mind.

"...shop the perimeter of the store..."

SAVE MONEY: Dietary intake that is lowfat, low-sugar, and high fiber is usually less expensive than a normal American high-fat diet. Turkey and chicken cost a lot less than red meats. Fresh vegetables and fruits cost less than already prepared frozen side dishes. Commercial baked items usually cost more than homemade lowfat cookies, cakes, and desserts.

A money-saving idea is to shop the perimeter (outer portion) of the store—where the fresh foods are located. The interior (center) aisles tend to carry the higher priced, highly processed, more fat and preservatives, and less fiber foods. You might need to selectively venture into the contraband areas to get whole grain cereals and pasta.

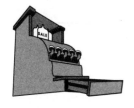

You may be surprised how far your food budget goes (as well as how much more nutritional it is) when you eliminate junk foods, fat-laden steaks and roasts, pies, cakes, and syrup-packed fruits from your shopping list. When you reduce costly meat and fish to healthier 100- or 200-calorie servings, you'll find your meat dishes making twice as many meals as they did in the past.

READ FOOD LABELS: Ignorance is bliss. Many products contain moderate amounts of sugars and/or fats. Don't assume a diet frozen dinner is lowfat. Many lite, lean, slim, or low-calorie dinners might be under 300 calories, but *they may also contain a lot of fat grams*. Check the label fat content and if over 9 grams of fat (some can have up to 20 grams or more), put it back on the shelf. Always check labels for the most nutritional products and for ones with the longest expiration dates.

"...lite might refer to serving size, sodium content, color..."

The Nutrition, Labeling and Education Act of 1990 will govern product labels over the next few years. Its dietary guidelines will assume a hypothetical daily intake of 2,000 calories (generally too many for someone wishing to reduce their weight). Until then, realize there is a lot of discrepancy in advertising terms being used. Lower-fat, slim, lean, or lite might be only empty claims. For example, *lite* might refer to serving size, sodium content, color, or fat content. Lite cream cheese has 5 fat grams per ounce, half the 10 fat grams of regular cream cheese. This still amounts to 40 fat grams (360 calories from fat) in an 8 ounce package.

The Food and Drug Administration (FDA) requires package labeling and health claims to be based on *realistic-size portions*. Unfortunately, this same standard doesn't apply to the poultry, meat, and dairy industries which operate under the U.S. Department of Agriculture (USDA). This is why a can of FDA-regulated vegetable soup might *appear* to have more fat than a can of USDA-regulated chicken soup.

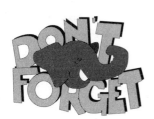

Labels such as *'cholesterol free'* can be confusing too. This is a trick used by some manufacturers to make you think an item is also 'fat free', which is not always the case. Even though cholesterol only comes from animal products, some plant products contain saturated fats that can raise our bad (LDL) cholesterol levels. Common ones in this category include palm and palm kernel oil, hydrogenated oil, cocoa butter, and coconut oil. Besides limiting these, other items to be limited contain things such as egg and egg-yolk solids; whole-milk solids; milk chocolate; shortening; lard; butter; and vegetable and partially hydrogenated vegetable oil.

Ingredients are listed on the labels from greatest amount to least amount. The product is probably okay if most ingredients are acceptable and *only one* unacceptable item appears in very low quantities (near the bottom of ingredient label). Look for high sodium, sugar, and fat contents (especially under their other names) and be aware that any series of items in brackets may be in that particular product.

Also carefully scrutinize the *91% fat free* processed luncheon meats as they may be labeled *fat by weight*, not by calories. Translated into calories, fats may actually be greater than 50% of the item.

DAIRY: Avoid whole milk and whole milk products. Since it contains from 3.5 to 4% fat (by weight), this translates into 50% of milk's calories coming from fat (mostly the unhealthier saturated kind). Use skim milk and low or

"Skip creamy salad dressings."

non-fat cheeses. Good choices for frozen desserts include lowfat yogurt, sorbet, fruit ices, sherbet and some ice milks.

DELI: Selections here should be fresh vegetables like tomatoes, cucumbers or sprouts, broccoli, mushrooms, peppers, or cauliflower. You can add garbanzos or other beans, peas or seeds for extra flavor and nutrition. Cider vinegar, lemon juice, or no-fat dressings are the best. You might also select lean roast beef, extra-lean ham, or baked turkey breast for a quick take-home meal. Don't overlook fish (usually in a nearby section) which is rich in omega-3 polyunsaturated fat that has been shown to help lower bad (LDL) cholesterol and blood triglyceride levels.

Avoid the prepared pasta, potato, or fruit salads made with mayonnaise or whipping cream. Watch even *mustard potato salad* as some contain egg yolks and mayonnaise. Skip creamy salad dressings. Avoid organ meats, brisket, and other high-fat meats.

Substitutions

The optimum dietary intake to achieve and maintain a healthy body, best energy levels, and your target weight is one which is based upon a variety of foods. You should be pleased to know that this is finally a program you can continue indefinitely. The days of agonizing over food sacrifices will be over. You can literally be set free to enjoy a world of good taste and good nutrition, all through simple substitutions and modifications.

"The optimum dietary intake ...based upon a variety of foods."

We are very fortunate to be living in the times we are. Just a few years ago, there were not nearly as many new, good tasting, lowfat and fat-free foods as there are now to replace the conventional high-fat ones. Almost every day, new ones seem to appear on the store shelves. Start slow and try substituting one or two low- or no-fat items at a time to help make changes gradually and prevent the psychological feeling of depravation and self-sacrifice. It will also help you know where to modify the recipe in the future if things don't turn out right the first time.

Many standard recipes use more salt, sugar, or fat than necessary. Try using half the amount of sugar listed. Why not use two egg whites instead of one whole egg? You can use lime or lemon juice and herbs to season vegetables, meats, or salads instead of butter. Instead of marinating fish, poultry, and meat in oil-based marinades, try ones using low-sodium soy sauce, lemon juice, wine, well-seasoned broth, or herb-flavored vinegar. Cream cheese can be replaced with Neufchatel cheese which is similar in taste and texture and has fewer calories.

Choose cooking methods that don't add additional fats to your foods, such as steaming, boiling, poaching, broiling, microwaving, dry roasting, or baking. Sautéing with butter, margarine, and oil can be replaced with a non-stick pan coated with spray vegetable oil pan coating (e.g. PAM), liquid Butter Buds, wine, or chicken broth. These fats can also be replaced in recipes with applesauce, corn syrup, or liquid Butter Buds. However, if oil is the only liquid in the recipe, try 1/2 non-fat milk and 1/2 applesauce to maintain moistness. In baking, substitute corn syrup in place of oil as this will maintain moist texture in combination with flour, sugar, and egg substitutes.

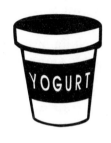

Skim milk can substitute for milk in many cases, and evaporated skim milk can replace cream in some recipes. Sour cream needed for baking? Why not try plain non-fat yogurt instead? Always try to select the *incomplete* mixes that allow you to add the oils and fats—once more giving control of fats to you for appropriate substitution. This can allow you to reduce fat in recipes from a third to a half. A cake mix requiring oil can be modified by using polyunsaturated oil at only two-thirds the amount called for while adding water to make up the additional one-third.

"You may find something better or with less fats..."

If attempting to lower weight, select diet foods whenever possible and check the calorie makeup of food on the package label carefully. Watch loosely used terms such as *lite* which can refer to color, portion size, or calorie content. Remember the goal is to do small things consistently rather than large things inconsistently.

The lists of substitutions can go on and on. In fact, they do and so we will list some possible substitutions below. Realize that these are just suggestions and not the only possible alternatives. You may find something better or with less fats and calories than the ones we have listed. Be inventive. This can be a very healthy mental exercise. For those of us that aren't that inventive, thank goodness for the good lowfat, low-calorie cookbooks on the market—try some!

> **FICTION:** It is necessary to spend one's lifetime dieting in order to control weight.
> **FACT:** If we think in terms of *quantity* and *frequency* of eating certain items and learn to make substitutions that don't increase caloric intake, we can overcome the *forbidden food* and dieting concept and get into the pleasure of healthy, positive, intelligent eating.

The following is a list of some commonly used food items in bold print, followed by one or more suggested alternatives in normal print. Obviously, the intended use of the food item will influence the substitution. For example, if you are just eating an avocado plain, you could substitute anything for it. However, if you are making guacamole dip, substitutions will be severely limited. Many books suggesting lowfat alternatives are on the market and should be consulted if you run out of ideas. The alternative suggestions are *not necessarily* what I would always recommend; they just present lower calorie alternatives to the initial choices.

SUBSTITUTION SUGGESTIONS

angel-food cake, 2" piece— cantaloupe melon, 1/2

avocado—lowfat cottage cheese; fruit

bacon—lowfat Canadian bacon (or fewer pieces)

bacon bits—Grape Nuts; crushed melba toast; mushrooms

baked items (commercial)— homemade baked items or fat-free

beans, baked—green beans

beans, immature—navy or pinto beans

beans, lima—asparagus, Brussels sprouts

beef tenderloin—lean top round or flank steak

beer—non-alcoholic beverage (even *near-beer*)

bread, white— gluten bread; whole grain breads

bread with butter—whole wheat bread plain or with 1 tsp. jam

butter—low-calorie margarine; butter-flavor granules

butter on toast—apple butter or fruit preserves on toast

cake—angel-food cake

cereal, sugar, puffed or highly refined—whole grain cereal; cereal with bran

cereal, wheat bran, rice or corn flakes—puffed wheat or puffed rice cereals

cheese, American, Swiss, cream, cheddar, blue—no-fat or lowfat cheese (e.g. fat-free mozzarella and 'lite' ricotta)

cheese cake—angel-food cake; lowfat homemade baked item

chicken breast, fried—chicken breast, broiled, no skin

chips, potato or corn—plain popcorn or pretzels

chocolate—Lite fudge topping; toasted marshmallows; Nestle Premier white chocolate

chocolate chips—reduced amount (1/4 to 1/2 of recipe)

cocoa, all milk—cocoa, milk and water

coffee creamers, non-dairy— lowfat dried milk in coffee

coffee with cream and sugar— coffee black with artificial sweetener or evaporated skim milk

cold cuts, high fat—lowfat sandwich meats

condiments, high fat—lowfat condiments such as fruit sauces (cranberries, apples, etc.) horseradish, chutney, or sweet pickle relish

cookies—dietetic vanilla wafers; air-popped popcorn; rice cakes

corn, canned—cauliflower

cream, heavy—evaporated skim milk

cream cheese—Neufchatel cheese; Weight Watchers Cream Cheese; or blend of cottage cheese, yogurt, and lemon juice

cupcake with icing—plain cupcake

custard—low-calorie cookies; non-fat frozen yogurt

Danish pastry—lowfat homemade baked item

donut—whole wheat bread with 1 tsp. jam

duck, roasted—roasted chicken

eggs—egg whites; Egg Beaters

egg yolks—egg whites; discard every other yolk and substitute 1 tsp. oil for discarded yolk in recipes

eggs, scrambled—boiled or poached egg

fish sticks—broiled cod or swordfish (consider pollutants)

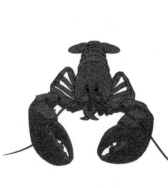

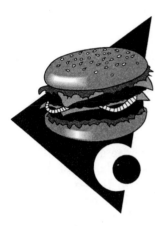

French fries—baked potato (plain or with lowfat yogurt)
fried items—baked, broiled, steamed items
fruit cake—individual fruits; fruit salad
fruit drink or fruit juice—fruit with the peel
fudge—dietetic vanilla wafers
granola or granola bars—any non-fat cereal
gravy—salsa
ground beef—ground skinless white turkey meat
ham—flounder or sole
hamburger—ground turkey or chicken; Healthy Choice ground beef
hamburger, broiled—lean broiled hamburger
hot dogs—sliced white meat turkey or lowfat hot dog (check *fat grams*)
ice cream—non-fat frozen yogurt or ice cream; banana (try it frozen); frozen fruit bars & pops; sherbet; ice milk; sorbet; air-popped popcorn (no butter)
juice, orange, 4 oz.—eat an orange
juice, prune, 8 oz.—tomato juice, 8 oz.
ketchup—homemade salsa (blend chopped fresh tomatoes, onions, lime juice, chilies, and spices)
lamb—fish; poultry
lamb chop, rib cut—roast lean leg of lamb
lard or solid vegetable shortening—corn, sunflower, or safflower oil
lobster meat with butter—lobster meat with lemon
loin roast—pot roast (round)

luncheon meats—lowfat turkey slices or water packed tuna
margarine, regular—diet margarine
mayonnaise—mustard or fat-free mayonnaise; dilute mayonnaise with nonfat yogurt, lemon juice, or vinegar
meat, red—chicken, turkey, or fish
meat loaf—club steak, flank steak
milk, whole—non-fat milk; skim milk; buttermilk
milkshake, chocolate malted—lemonade
muffin, plain—oat bran muffin
muffins or biscuits (commercial)—homemade or fat-free mixes
noodles cooked with oil, and butter added after draining—leave oil out of cooking water and don't add butter to steaming noodles
nuts—Grape Nuts cereal; rice wafers; or use 1/2 recipe amount
ocean perch, fried—baked or broiled bass
oil, butter, and margarine—applesauce, corn syrup, liquid butter-flavor granules, or non-stick sprays
oil in recipes—reduce by 1/3 to 1/2 and substitute extra water for missing oil
olives—pickles; carrot sticks; celery
oysters, fried—oysters on half-shell with low-calorie sauce (but consider hepatitis)
peanut butter—low sugar jelly
peanut butter and jelly sandwich—open face egg salad sandwich
peanuts, roasted—grapes; cereal without milk as a snack

peanuts, salted—apple, celery, or other crunchable food
peas, canned—spinach
pie, apple—small apple or citrus fruit
pie, blueberry—unsweetened blueberries
pie, cherry—whole cherries
pie, custard—small banana
pie, lemon meringue—flavored gelatin
pie, peach—whole peach
pie, rhubarb—cantaloupe
pork—lean pork tenderloin
pork chop—veal chop
pork roast—veal roast
pork sausage—lean ham
potato, fried—baked potato
potato, mashed—boiled potato
potato chips—baked potato with salsa; pretzels
pound cake—plums; low-calorie homemade cake without icing
prime rib—filet mignon
pudding, flavored—non-fat milk dietetic pudding
rice, white—brown rice or other legume
rump roast—rib roast
salad, chef, with oil dressing, mayonnaise or Russian, French, blue cheese or Roquefort dressing—chef salad with dietetic dressing or lemon juice
salad dressing—low-calorie, lowfat or oil-free salad dressing; fresh squeezed lemon juice; balsamic vinegar
salt—herbs, spices, and/or lemon or lime juice

sandwich, club—open face bacon and tomato sandwich
sauce, Alfredo or cream—marinara sauce (tomato based)
sausage—ground turkey
sauté with butter, margarine or oil—use wine, Butter Buds, or chicken broth
snack crackers—fat-free saltines
soda, regular—diet soda
soup, bean—beef noodle soup
soup, chicken noodle—split pea or bean soup
soup, cream of mushroom—vegetable soup
soup, creamed—chicken noodle soup; broth
soup, minestrone—beef bouillon
sour cream—blend of lemon juice, non-fat cottage cheese, and non-fat yogurt
sour cream in baking—plain non-fat yogurt
steak, T-bone—lean hamburger; flank steak
steak, porterhouse—club steak
succotash—spinach; squash
sugar—artificial sweetener
tortilla chips—melba toast; Guiltless Gourmet brand chips
tuna, canned—canned crabmeat
tuna, in oil—tuna in water
turkey with gravy—open face lean hamburger
veal—turkey cutlets
vegetable, low fiber—high fiber vegetable
walnuts—1/2 recipe amount of nuts
winter squash—summer squash

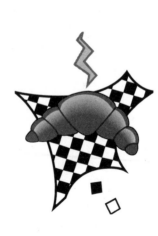

Mealtime Tips

Cooking

This section will summarize some cooking tips. Other suggestions for cooking may be found throughout this book, as well as in many fine lowfat, low-calorie cookbooks available in most bookstores.

Be aware that some foreign cooking terms may be actually translated **fat added**. *Au gratin* identifies a dish with cheese sauce. *Tempura* means *fried in butter*. *Sauté* signifies to *add butter*. Broiling may sound safe, and should be, unless the item is broiled in butter (e.g. restaurant seafood).

"Adapt recipes to use minimal fat and oil..."

Try sautéing foods such as garlic, onions, celery, and mushrooms in wine, vermouth, seasoned water, flavored vinegar, bouillon, or chicken stock instead of in oil, lard, shortening, margarine, or butter. Use no more than one tablespoon of oil or margarine if you elect not to substitute when sautéing.

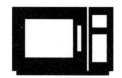

Adapt recipes to use minimal (or no) fat and oil and choose preparation methods that require minimal use of them such as baking, boiling, poaching, steaming, broiling, roasting, or microwaving—and discard the drippings. Vertical roasting of poultry reduces fats also. Always use a non-stick pan to cook with and coat it with a non-fat cooking spray (e.g. PAM) as needed.

Microwaving ground beef on paper towels seems to get rid of more fat that broiling, roasting, or pan frying it. You might be interested to know that microwaving certain foods may be healthful for reasons other than eliminating cooking oils and fats. Some studies have shown that microwaving conserves more B and C vitamins than conventional cooking.

Choose *incomplete* mixes that allow you to control the fat content, and use diet, tub, or squeeze margarines or unsaturated oils to complete them. Fats can also be controlled by cooking soups, chili, spaghetti sauce, and stews *the day before* and refrigerating them to make it easier to skim off the solidified fat that will accumulate.

"Avoid overcooking vegetables..."

Another way to save dietary fat is to *not* brown meat and vegetables together. Vegetables act like fat magnets or sponges and should be browned separately. Avoid overcooking vegetables as this depletes minerals, vitamins, and fiber benefits. Marinating food with tomato or onion soup, spices, lowfat beef broth, wine or lemon can replace the need for high fat content or frying to bring out delectable flavors.

Try to trim meat, poultry, and fish of all skin, fat, and bone before weighing and cooking. Partially freeze poultry and meat if you wish to trim excess fat and want to slice the meat thinly for stir-frying (with minimal oil or PAM). After cooking meat, especially ground meat or poultry, drain on a paper towel or colander and rinse with hot water to remove even more residual fat.

"...become aware of emotional food triggers..."

If cooking Italian, use marinara sauce instead of the Alfredo. Try leaving the oil out of the pasta cooking water and don't add the butter to the hot noodles as some recipes call for. You may add the sauce to help keep pasta from sticking.

Rice is another starch that people worry about sticking or clumping. Like the pasta, you don't have to add margarine or butter to add flavor or prevent sticking. Instead, add herbs and cook in tomato juice or flavored broth to add flavor with minimal calories.

Don't cook cream-based soups. Cook broth-based ones instead. If you need to, you can make your own *cream* soups by using vegetable purees, skim milk, or yogurt.

Easy on the salt shaker, especially during food preparation and cooking. Don't salt foods until you taste them, and then only if you have to. Try using the *powders* instead of the *salts* (e.g. garlic or celery powder) for variety. Better still, let each individual add their own salt at the table and limit your own intake as suggested.

Eating Meal

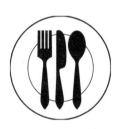

Your body needs *six* ingredients for balanced nutrition. These can be classified as *water*, *macronutrients*—protein, carbohydrate, and fat, and *micronutrients*—vitamins and minerals. The key to having a nutritional balance of these ingredients when you eat is to have food variety. Avoid getting into the *same thing* every meal rut (e.g. tuna for lunch everyday) as this may become boring very quickly. Variety keeps your weight management program appealing and successful, and it keeps you out of the *diet* frame of mind.

"Practice eating slowly..."

Don't forget the importance of a *food-mood* diary in which you make note of your emotions and moods each time you find yourself eating. This helps you to become aware of emotional food triggers, which in turn can allow you to substitute another activity for food.

As you eat, take the time to enjoy what you are doing. Practice eating slowly, chewing your food more times, and enjoying—REALLY ENJOYING—the food and the oasis of time in your day.

Realize that food has many flavors and tastes and savor each one before swallowing it (not shoveling it). Putting the fork down between each bite as you are doing this and not being distracted by other activities (e.g. TV or reading) can also help you practice nutrition enjoyment and life appreciation. Use this time to give thanks for the positive aspects of your life and health. Try to discuss only positive things during the meal, not negative.

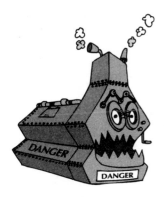

The art of eating slowly is something so many of us need to develop. Besides not taking the time to reflect (as mentioned above), eating quickly doesn't allow our stomach to tell our brain that it is full and that the body should be satisfied, so we miss an important signal for fullness. Hunger can take up to twenty minutes to be offset by a meal, so plan time in your day to make your meal last at least this long. Watch the clock if you have to or get up and take a stretch break during the meal. Otherwise, you will probably eat more than if you were eating more slowly.

Food should be chewed well. It's hard to imagine how people can truly enjoy food that is swallowed almost whole. Chewing longer and more thoroughly allows you to become even more aware of the food you are eating and sensitive to its taste.

Cut food into smaller pieces and take smaller bites. You can chew each bite twenty times or so and don't use fingers to feed yourself, only utensils (consider chopsticks to slow down). Some studies have shown overweight people have a tendency to take larger mouthfuls of food than thin individuals. Many folks are not even aware of this. Limiting yourself on quantity will be easier if you use smaller pieces and take smaller bites. It truly is amazing how satisfying relatively small portions of food can be.

Don't reload your fork or spoon until the previous mouthful is finished. Actually get up from the table for several minutes and stretch, walk around, pour more water, etc. to help stretch the eating experience. A true gourmet enjoys eating and you can too!

You may wish to start meals with a high carbohydrate food, such as bean or noodle soup, bread without butter, or a pasta appetizer. This may help reduce your craving for fat as the meal progresses and could help you steer clear of a high-fat dessert.

"...don't exclude daily vegetable intake..."

If you have a salad, flavor it with basil, parsley, or cilantro, or select lemon juice, seasoned vinegar, or other herb/spice blends without salt for dressings. However, don't exclude daily vegetable intake by substituting salads for them. Choose steamed vegetables more often than salad when possible. Steaming ruptures the starch molecule in the food and makes it more satisfying to some than just the fiber of a salad.

Limit sauces on vegetables and other foods whenever you can. Tomato or wine-based sauces usually contain less fat than those made from cream, eggs, cheese, sour cream, or butter.

So much of our eating is *pattern eating*. If we break the cycle, sometimes this will allow us to venture in a new direction. This becomes very important in behavior modification and adopting new eating behaviors and a healthy lifestyle. The following are a few tips to help control eating habits at the table:

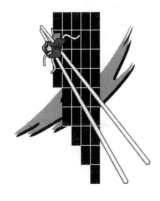

- Put food on a smaller plate (e.g. 7" instead of 9"), which may help portion sizes look larger.
- Eat with a salad or dessert fork (or chopsticks).
- Pamper yourself by changing to a new table setting (plates and silverware).
- Avoid serving food *boarding house style* with it in large dishes that remain on the table. Keep the extra portions off the table and no second helpings (this could make another meal tomorrow).
- You don't have to clean your plate, leave some food. Give the extra to the dog or put it immediately into the trash or disposal. A second on the lips—forever on the hips.
- Make meals last at least 20 minutes (the time required for the brain to register that you have eaten).
- Have family members clean off their own plates. This will reduce your temptation.

Portion Control

Be aware of serving sizes. Large commercial food institutions that process foods know the importance of portion control in relation to their food costs. You should be just as familiar with its importance in relation to your weight and health costs.

Just selecting lowfat foods will not give you the weight management freedom to consume 4,000 calories a day and maintain control of your weight. There may be virtually no fat in two bags of jelly beans, ten dietetic cookies, or two pints of non-fat frozen yogurt—but don't expect eating all this to help you lose weight and be healthy. Use common sense and good judgment (as well as healthy food choices).

"The best diet foods may be some you are currently eating..."

Don't just eat cottage cheese and canned tuna to try to lose weight. Re-train yourself to eat smaller (diet) portions of foods you already eat. The best *diet* foods may be some you are currently eating—just smaller portions. It's been said before but bears repeating again—there are no forbidden foods. Just watch quantity and frequency of consuming the obviously *problem* ones.

You can even make small portions seem larger. Large amounts of food on large platters appear smaller than they really are. Of course, the reverse is true too. Why not obtain plates moderately smaller than the ones you have now and use them consistently? Spreading the food out on a plate rather than piling it up also gives the sensation that there is more than there actually is.

Realize serving foods *family style*, in large pass-around dishes, encourages larger portions and second helpings. A better method is to place appropriately sized portions on individual plates.

Prayer, Reflection, Thankfulness

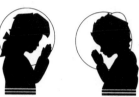

The way we live and the way we eat have potentially immense consequences for the quality of life and path we take. When we take time to be thankful for the very food that sustains us, we touch on something very basic in all of life itself—that food and life are precious. Not everyone may have the opportunity to sit and enjoy food and nourishment with family and friends. This is a precious commodity that many hungry people of the world can only dream about—don't take it for granted.

"...expressing our sense of gratitude..."

When we say grace, we are expressing our sense of gratitude and kinship with life. It is not so much the words we say as the state of mind we evoke that is important. Think how precious it is to have a moment to look inward into our very being, and slow down, relax, and block out the day's worries and hectic schedule while we give thanks for the food we are about to receive. We can reflect upon our community, our country, and our world and sense a bond with other life on this planet that may be sitting down at that very moment to eat and reflect. Our sincere spirit of thankfulness can put us in touch with someone higher than ourselves and can help us focus our lives and give purpose and direction to who we are and where we are going. This is an important part of our day also.

Soups

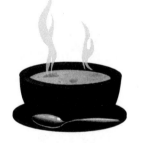

Soups are a good start to a meal as they can be very tasty and quite filling. For some, tomato soup may supply more appetite suppression than other kinds. When eaten slowly and soon enough before the main meal, soup can help curb appetite so that you can eat less during the main and subsequent courses of the meal. A large pot of soup can be made up ahead of time and divided into smaller containers for freezing or later use.

"Soups are a good start to a meal..."

If purchasing commercially prepared soups, check the labels for fats and sodium. Try to select those low in sodium and with 5 fat grams or less per serving. Choose clear soups such as bouillon or broth (however, these can be high in sodium).

Desserts

Have you noticed that *desserts* is *stressed* spelled backwards? This can definitely be one of the more stressful aspects of proper eating, yet desserts are one of the easiest parts of our dietary modifications to make lowfat. Once again, *modification and substitution* become the cornerstone

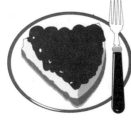

"Avoid high fat desserts..."

of building new eating habits. As you learn to make simple changes the possibilities become endless. Try lowfat substitutions and you could be in for a *sweet* surprise. You may be amazed how far simple things like Egg Beaters, Butter Buds, lowfat cottage cheese, buttermilk, plain yogurt, applesauce, and artificial sweeteners will go. You can even substitute cocoa for chocolate in certain recipes.

Choose lowfat cookies and cakes made with canola, sunflower, or safflower oil. Try angel food cake and other lowfat desserts, such as sorbet, frozen lowfat yogurt, lowfat custard, fruit salad, and fresh fruits. Use yogurt in place of cream. You can even use it mixed with a touch of honey to make a great lowfat fruit dessert dressing. Make your own fresh fruit dessert with sliced bananas, diced pears and apples, grapes, tangerine sections, and a dash of orange juice concentrate. One-half cup is about 70 calories.

Avoid high-fat desserts such as pastries, cheesecake, fruit pies, and hard cheeses. As you are modifying similar desserts, try cutting down on sugar (by 1/3 to 1/2 the recipe amount) in cakes, cookies, and quick breads. Heighten the effect of sweetness in low-sugar desserts by using sweet spices such as cinnamon, nutmeg, ginger, and vanilla. Go easy on bitter or sour ingredients such as lemon.

Leftovers

"...prepare only what you need to eat..."

The best way to avoid leftovers is to prepare only what you *need* to eat at each meal (especially the appropriate quantity). If the sight of uneaten food is a cue for you to overeat, plan ahead of time what to do with leftovers. When the meal is finished, clear the table immediately. Put any high-calorie leftovers in difficult to open, opaque or frosted containers (or foil) in the back of the refrigerator. At least wrap them up tightly to discourage nibbling. Consider turning off the refrigerator light bulb to make tempting foods harder to see.

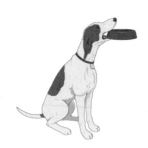

You may also feed leftovers to the pets or put them directly into the garbage or disposal. Realize that pets do not need a lot of high fat table food either. Also, don't make the mistake of allowing tomorrow's meal to become tonight's late-night snack. All non-perishable, tempting foods should be placed at the very back of the pantry or on a top shelf requiring a kitchen stool to reach them. The harder temptation is, the easier it becomes to avoid it.

Get out of the mind set of having to 'clean your platter'. Try leaving some food on your plate *every* time you have a meal. You may have grown up in a family where leaving food on the plate was considered unacceptable. How many times did you hear about "all the starving people in China"? It probably never occurred to those telling you this that those starving Chinese could never be helped by an overweight American who overeats. It only takes a few extra bites each meal to add up to several extra unwanted pounds in a year or so.

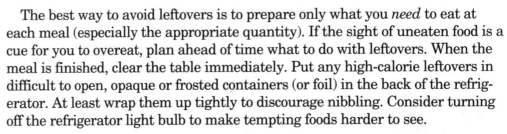

Snacking

Snacking, in the usual sense of the word, is really an unnecessary part of good nutrition and should be a habit that is modified. However, if we are to be totally realistic, the fact remains that it will occur from time to time. The intelligent thing is to know how to snack appropriately and in as healthy a manner as possible.

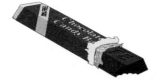

Before you begin to feel deprived, once again realize that there is no food that cannot occasionally be eaten (e.g. dessert, cake, chocolate, wine, etc.). It is the quantity and frequency that is crucial (but don't abuse this privilege and your body).

"Eat problem food in a controlled setting..."

Eat *problem* foods in a controlled setting—such as in front of other people—so that you will be aware of how much you are really eating. A half gallon of ice cream is easier to gulp down at home than in public. Set a limit and stick to it, and of course it wouldn't hurt to *not have* ready-to-eat snack foods around the house.

Some simple guidelines for snacking are to avoid bingeing, as it is usually some internal need *other than* true hunger (look for emotional triggers and substitute non-food activities as countermeasures). Try not to snack while preparing dinner or when the urge first hits you during the day. Find something to keep your hands and mind busy instead, such as walking the dog, playing games with the kids, practicing the piano or guitar, knitting or cross-stitching, etc.

If you eat out of boredom, find some new hobby or interest that gets you away from temptation (even consider adult education courses). Snack on lowfat foods like pretzels, air-popped corn, dry whole grain cereals, or apples.

If you *plan* snacks as part of your day, then once again you will be in control of them because you will decide what, when, and where they will be. Plan for occasional special treats, important weekends and other special occasions rather than being *surprised* and having to make spur-of-the-moment decisions.

- Candy is something that has many options, especially if watching calories and fats. Try to stick to hard candies such as clear lollipops, sour balls, lemon drops, or peppermints.
- Check labels carefully on everything, especially potato and corn chip snacks. Many *lite* varieties may be high in sodium, fat, and calories. Try to avoid buttered popcorn, Cheetos, regular potato chips, chocolate, corn or tortilla chips, and carob bars.
- Choose lowfat vegetable or noodle soups and avoid the creamy ones. Some types of cup-a-soup are also okay. Be sure to watch the sodium content.

"Use lowfat muffins..."

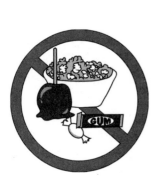

"...popcorn ...season with herbs or spices..."

- Cut down on baked goods made with lard, palm kernel or coconut oil, or shortening, as well as those deep fried in fats/oils, such as doughnuts.
- Dried fruit can contain up to 70% sugar by weight. This is similar to the amount in some candies.
- Eat single-crust (open-face) pies instead of typical two-crust pies. You can also eat the filling from pie and leave the crust (containing most of the fats) behind.
- Freeze seedless grapes, banana chunks, pears, melons, or peaches for cool, refreshing snack treats (especially nice during the summer months).
- Graham crackers, raisin biscuits, popcorn cakes or rice cakes can be lowfat treats when you have the munchies.
- Nuts and seeds are good protein sources and are a significant source of fiber and vitamin E but also tend to be high in fat (though largely unsaturated fat). Chestnuts are the exception as one ounce has 64 calories and less than a gram of fat. Limit intake of nuts if concerned about excess calorie intake. Avoid those roasted (which actually means *fried*) in palm, palm kernel, or coconut oil as these are saturated fats. Dry-roasted nuts are not appreciably lower in fat than regular roasted nuts because nuts are so high in fat to begin with.
- Raisins can be a quick, on-the-go treat but can give you a lot of calories if you eat a lot of them.
- Select fresh and dried fruits and vegetables. Fresh fruits and vegetables like apples, oranges, and carrot sticks are colorful lowfat, ready-to-eat snacks.
- Try plain popcorn (beware *light* varieties) and season with herbs or spices without salt. You would have to consume almost two quarts of plain, unbuttered popcorn to get the same amount of calories as in one ounce of potato chips (about 15 chips). Regular popcorn cooked in a microwave has about 1/3 the calories and fat of commercial microwavable brands. Air-popped, unbuttered popcorn has only about three percent of its calories from fat, compared to 76 percent of a peanuts' calories. Place plain popcorn in a brown paper bag and fold over the top, put it in the center of the microwave, and cook three minutes or so on the *high* setting. Don't add oil or other ingredients until after cooking. Instead of using oil or fat, spray popcorn lightly with vegetable coating and then sprinkle with onion or chili powder, curry, or cinnamon for an alternative taste treat.
- Try raw vegetables with a dip made from plain yogurt seasoned with herbs instead of sour cream. You might also try the yogurt for sour cream substitution in some salad dressings too.
- Use lowfat muffins, jelly beans, fruit rolls, lowfat cookies, and frozen fruit bars or popsicles.

Dining Out

More and more of us are eating away from home. According to the National Restaurant Association, Americans spend 43 percent of their food budget eating out. Many of these meals tend to be high in fat, low in fiber, and not nutritionally balanced. If you dine out more than once a week, it is no longer a special treat that justifies *blowing your diet*. You need to eat as you would at home: sensibly, healthfully, and making lowfat selections. Part of this American trend may be that we have geared our social life towards eating and drinking events. This needs to be modified to allow us to focus on activities, such as skating, dancing, bowling, or spectator sports (without the hot dog and cheese nachos).

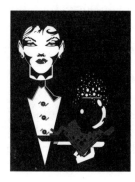

Be selective where you go to eat and you pick the restaurant, if possible. Eat at the same restaurant regularly so that you are familiar with and feel confident in ordering from their menu. Cafeterias are convenient since they have a moderate amount of food choices and you can see the sizes of the portions being served. If someone else selects where you will be eating, don't hesitate to *call ahead* and ask about healthy choices on their menu or if something could be prepared *to-order*. The chef may be able to prepare lowfat sauce or a lowfat dish for you in place of their regular fare. This may just require preparation without butter or oil.

"...don't starve yourself prior to eating out..."

Try to save excess calories but don't starve yourself prior to eating out or going to the social event. Eat sensible lowfat choices all day, but do eat. Otherwise, you will arrive ravenous and can easily overeat before you get a *full feeling*. You may find eating a small, lowfat snack (fruit, soup, etc.) prior to going out helps keep you in control of the situation.

Once you arrive, position yourself away from the food tables. Have salad dressing *on the side*, if at all. Begin the meal with hot, clear soup and avoid the cream soups. During the meal, eat moderately and avoid fried and sauce-laden dishes. Ask the waitperson what you want to know, especially about items you are unsure about. Ask how the food is prepared and what is in the sauce or soup. Order seafood, lean beef entrees, and vegetables *plain* or *dry*, with no added oils, salt, or monosodium glutamate (MSG). Request white meat if eating turkey or chicken (1/2 the calories of dark meat), and be sure to remove the skin before eating it. Why not skip the sweets and pastries at the end of the meal and settle for coffee or fresh fruit. A glass of wine is fine but why not satisfy your thirst with water or mineral water.

"Practicing ahead of time will also help..."

Practicing ahead of time will also help you modify your eating habits. Become familiar with foods averaging less than 30% calories from fats. Pre-plan your food choices mentally at home or before the social event. Practice measuring foods at home as this will allow you to be familiar with appropriate portion sizes that fall within your eating guidelines. Then, if servings are too large, you can eat half of it or share it with a partner. It's okay to leave food on the plate or ask for a *take home* bag.

ON THE SIDE: Try to get salad dressings, butter, and sauces served on the side. This allows you to regulate your intake of these typically high-fat items and puts you in control. Dip your fork in the salad dressing, then spear the salad and you still get the flavor without using so much dressing. You may also take small packets of non-fat dressing with you in a purse or pocket. Send the butter or condiment back to the kitchen if you can't stay away from it.

DINNER PARTIES: If you find these a problem, eat low-calorie, high bulk items or clear soup before attending. Even if out of town, you can usually get fruits at a grocery or convenience store and have those before the meal. While at the party, eat slowly, enjoying the atmosphere or conversation. While others are on their second helpings, you can still be on your first.

"...eat slowly, enjoying the atmosphere..."

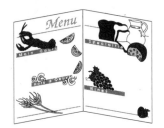

SHARING: It is becoming more acceptable to share meals and desserts with others in your party. Order one dessert and several forks and share the calories. Several bites will keep you from feeling deprived and reassure you that you are eating, not sacrificing. You could even skip the dessert and go out for a non-fat frozen yogurt after the meal.

MENUS: Some restaurants have other selections besides just what you see on the menu. For example, in today's health conscious society, some restaurants might make you a *vegetable plate* from several selections, even though it may not be listed on the menu. You can usually stick to simple things with great success, such as baked potatoes, salads, spaghetti, rice, or steamed vegetables.

SCALE WATCHING: The pounds shown on the bathroom scales the next morning may not be a true reflection of your eating the night before. Several pounds increase can sometimes be from fluid retention due to more highly seasoned and salted food that what you may ordinarily consume. Hopefully, it was not due to a large dietary indiscretion. Continue to drink adequate fluid and you should shed this excess fluid retention.

In an effort to help you develop your own guidelines, I will offer suggestions for a meal and then offer suggestions for selected types of restaurants. Your choices may differ, but remember your ultimate health and weight goals and make selections accordingly.

THE MEAL

BEVERAGES: Hot or cold teas and coffees (decaffeinated or regular), mineral waters, and artificially sweetened carbonated beverages may be selected. Use sugar substitutes to sweeten. Skim milk is preferred to whole milk when needed.

APPETIZERS: Choose hot, clear soups or broths, consommé, bouillon, dill pickles, celery sticks, or radishes. Hot hors d'oeuvres are usually fried, stuffed or wrapped in high-fat bacon or pastry. It's okay to eat raw vegetables with salsa instead of dip. Crab, shrimp, pretzels, or fresh fruit might provide alternative selections to this portion of a social event. A little planning here goes a long way towards calorie control.

BREADS and **CEREALS:** Several restaurants will make hot cereal to order and also carry cold, non-sugared cereals. Adding skim milk and even fresh fruit can be a healthy thing to do. Try whole-grained bread or toast without margarine or butter. A teaspoon of jam on the toast is a good butter alternative.

SALADS: A good selection could be raw vegetable salads without dressing or with it on the side. Darker green lettuce tends to be best. Lemon juice, flavored vinegar, or lowfat salad dressings can be used to compliment the salad. Beware commercial croutons as they are loaded with oil. Substitute crumbled melba toast in your salad for crunch without a lot of calories.

ENTREE: Fish or poultry that hasn't been fried or broiled with butter are healthy selections. Leave off gravies and fancy sauces (or serve on the side). Trim all visible fat from meat and remove skin from poultry prior to eating (preferably prior to cooking).

VEGETABLES: Try to get them boiled, steamed, stewed, or baked. Avoid the cream or cheese sauces.

"...split a high-calorie dessert with a friend..."

POTATOES: Steamed, boiled, baked, or mashed present quite a variety of selections. Toppings could include salsa, lowfat salad dressing or cottage cheese, or yogurt. Sweet potatoes are acceptable if not candied.

FATS: Try to skip regular salad dressings, fried foods, lunch meats, pork, beef, cheese, sour cream, whole milk, margarine, and butter.

DESSERTS: Fresh fruits, flavored ices, sorbets, and sherbets are refreshing. After dinner black coffee might provide caffeine but few calories. You can split a high-calorie dessert with a friend or spouse.

RESTAURANTS

DELI: Select greens and skip prepared potato, pasta, or fruit salads made with whipping cream or mayonnaise. Mustard potato salad may be misleading (it may contain mayonnaise and egg yolks). Flavored vinegar or lemon juice are the best salad dressings; leave off the creamy ones. Choose lean roast beef, lean or fat-free ham, or baked turkey breasts. Add garbanzos or other beans, peas or seeds for extra flavor. Load up on the fresh vegetables, such as cucumbers, tomatoes, peppers, cauliflower, broccoli, or mushrooms.

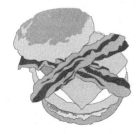

FAST FOODS: Many fast food establishments offer a grilled chicken sandwich. If you get it on a multigrain bun without sauce or mayonnaise, it can make for a good choice. You can usually find baked or broiled fish somewhere in your neighborhood. Use lemon for flavoring on it instead of butter. Some fast food restaurants offer salad bars and baked potatoes, but beware of the luncheon meats, cole slaw, cottage cheese (usually the whole milk variety), bacon, eggs, pasta salads, and high-calorie dressings at these salad bars. Watch the commercial croutons, nuts and seeds as these can add extra calories and fats.

CONTINENTAL: Look for the pasta and seafood selections that you can request to be prepared lowfat. Avoid veal, pork, beef, rack of lamb, or duck.

STEAK: Have the bread without butter. Many offer seafood and chicken selections. Some have pasta dishes also. If you need an appetizer, the shrimp cocktail may be lower calorie than some of the other selections. As a last resort, eat *lean* meat cooked *well done* to keep calories lower.

"The best advice is to plan ahead..."

CHINESE: Usually a good place for noodles and vegetable dishes. Ask to have food prepared without oil or fat. Don't eat anything fried with a crust. Avoid duck, pork, or beef, and instead select chicken and seafood dishes that aren't fried. If you do order fried rice, try to pick chicken or shrimp over pork.

BARBECUE: Chicken offers the lowest fat choice compared to pork, beef, and sausage. Order white meat chicken (1/2 the calories of dark) and remove the skin. Eat plain whole wheat bread and avoid the corn bread or muffins. Unbuttered corn and green beans are fine. A baked potato plain or with Butter Buds or diet dressing might be another selection.

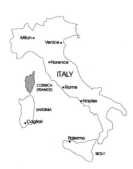

ITALIAN: Select pasta dishes with marinara sauce, not Alfredo or creamy or butter sauce. Choose seafood or chicken and avoid lamb, beef, or veal. Plain bread without garlic and butter is okay. If selecting pizza, ask for half the usual amount of cheese and get vegetable toppings instead of meat ones. Pan pizzas usually contain a lot of oil (and calories) in the crust. Order the flavored ices for dessert instead of cheesecake or high calorie after-dinner drinks.

MEXICAN: The first temptation to overcome is the chips with sauce. If you can't pass them up, at least set a limit (10 or 15), break them, and eat them slowly, enjoying each bite. Better still, order corn or flour tortillas and eat them (no butter) with the sauce instead of the chips. Eat as much hot sauce as you want but avoid the chili con queso. Usually chicken fajitas (cooked without oil) are the lowest fat menu item. Order them with lettuce and tomato on the side instead of the usual high-fat setup of guacamole, sour cream, and cheese.

The better Mexican restaurants will be able to make enchiladas, tacos, and burritos to your preferences. Any chicken or seafood dish not cooked in cream sauce or butter might also be a reasonable selection. Skip the fried sopapillas, egg dishes, and cream soups. Try to avoid the refried beans (may contain lard) by ordering double rice instead.

MOVIES: Though not a restaurant, some suggestions may be in order for this high calorie eating spot. The best advice is to plan ahead and treat yourself to a sensible dessert before going to the movies. You might also wish to take a healthy snack with you, such as a small can of fruit juice, raisins, dry roasted nuts, or cooked at home popcorn. The junk food and hot dogs at the counter are dietary disasters waiting to happen.

Travelers Tips

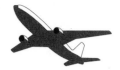

How Business Travelers Can Eat Healthfully On The Road*

When you're on a short vacation, eating high-fat, high-sodium foods for a few days probably won't cause you many problems. But for those business travelers who spend a lot of time on the road, combining too much high-fat, high-sodium food with too little exercise over the months and years can be disastrous.

"Be wary of the breakfast special..."

Getting a quick, nutritious breakfast is difficult when you're traveling. If you eat out, choose foods such as pancakes (short stack) and eat them with syrup or preserves and no added butter or margarine. Other possibilities: whole-grain toast or bagels (plain or spread lightly with margarine or jam), hot cereal with fresh berries or fruit, and lowfat milk. Be wary of the *breakfast special*, which usually contains foods that are no bargain for your body.

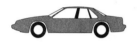

Consider taking breakfast items with you from home or picking them up at a local store when you arrive at your destination. The possibilities include whole-grain, ready-to-eat cereal, banana, and skim or 1 percent milk kept cold in a hotel ice bucket; nonfat yogurt with fruit; or even graham crackers with fruit and skim milk. If your only choice is a continental breakfast, stick with the bran or corn muffins and avoid the doughnuts and pastries.

Midday can be a difficult time for many health- and weight-conscious business travelers, since time and choices may be limited. Happily, fast-food establishments are offering more and more healthful choices for their patrons. Among them: a grilled skinless chicken-breast sandwich, a roast beef sandwich, or a regular-size hamburger with lettuce, tomato, and mustard. Try a side salad with diet dressing or a baked potato that isn't soaked with butter, instead of fries.

"Some national chains offer soup-and-salad..."

Another way to get your daily ration of vegetables is to choose the salad bar. Stick with plenty of the veggies and add small amounts of the protein choices, such as tuna, egg white, kidney or garbanzo beans, cottage cheese, and boiled ham or turkey. Beware of the mayonnaise-laden salads dripping with fat and calories. Order juice, milk, iced tea, diet soda, or water, rather than a shake or regular soda. Remember that a hot dog from a stand contains twice the fat and salt of a hamburger.

Some national chains offer soup-and-salad or soup-and-sandwich specials at lunch. Be sure to ask for salad dressings on the side and no added mayonnaise on the bread.

If you prefer deli sandwiches, stick with sliced turkey or chicken breast, boiled ham, tuna, hummus (Middle Eastern chick-pea spread), or lean roast beef, rather than cold-cut subs, BLT's, or Reuben sandwiches. You can make a big difference in fat and calories by eliminating mayonnaise and cheese from your sandwiches. If possible, try to get less of the above fillings and then fill the sandwich with vegetables: lettuce, tomato, sprouts, or cucumber slices.

What about pizza as another alternative? Stick to pizza with vegetables and skip the fat-laden meats and extra cheese. Be sure to order pizza in the appropriate portion, so there isn't a temptation to overeat. Salad is a good starter while you're waiting for the pizza to arrive.

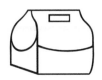

If you're traveling by car, it certainly is possible to carry along a cooler packed with healthy lunch items. This can give more variety for lunches for the first couple of days on the road. Your cooler could include healthful leftovers, lowfat cottage cheese, three-bean salad, or sardines in mustard with lowfat crackers.

"...avoid the all-you-can-eat places."

When it comes time for dinner, avoid the *all you can eat* places. Good choices for restaurant dining are places where foods are individually prepared. Even though French restaurants have the reputation for being all cream and eggs, you can easily get broiled fish or seafood with sauces on the side, fresh vegetables, or salad, by making your desires known to the waiter. Be sure to ask how foods are prepared, because sometimes the description on the menu can be deceiving.

Ethnic restaurants that can provide good dinner choices are Indian, Italian, Japanese, and Afghan, among others. Choose broiled seafood, lean grilled kebobs, or spaghetti with clam sauce or red sauce (avoid cream sauces). Of course, *portion size is a major factor*. Try to get a three- or four-ounce portion (about the size and thickness of the palm of your hand or the size of a deck of cards). If the portion you're served is too large, ask for a doggie bag; you can put the leftovers in your hotel ice bucket and have them for breakfast or lunch the next day.

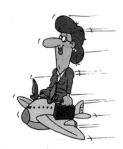

If you're a frequent flier, don't forget to order a special meal. Depending on the airline you choose, a variety of special options are available, from a seafood or fruit plate to low calorie or low cholesterol. These special meals can get your trip off to a healthy start. Usually, you must order them at least 24 hours in advance. The low-cholesterol breakfasts are especially good for saving on fat, cholesterol, and calories.

There are always those times on the road when we don't want to worry about fat and calories. It is probably OK to indulge yourself occasionally, as long as you get back to normal the next day. And take advantage of hotels that offer exercise facilities to burn off those extra calories.

Reprinted by permission, Nation's Business, *October 1990.*
Copyright © 1990, U.S. Chamber of Commerce.

Fast Foods

One survey reported that 40-50% of the calories in most fast food meals comes from fat. Since many *fast food* restaurants can therefore be translated *FAT food* restaurants, it may be difficult to eat healthy if you consume a lot of these foods.

It is estimated that fast food restaurants serve about 45.8 million people (a fifth of the American population) every day. Every second an estimated 200 people in the U.S. are served a hamburger...and the trend continues.

Listed below you will find some suggestions on how to select as lowfat and low-calorie as you can, given the aforementioned circumstances. You can also find tips elsewhere in this book, including the 'Travelers Tips' section.

BREAKFAST: Bran muffins and non-sugared cereals with lowfat milk are good choices. Biscuits and croissants are high in fat. Try the Burger King Bagel with cheese and egg or McDonald's Egg McMuffin as these might be lower fat selections than some other items. One of the worst choices is Burger King Croissan'wich with sausage, egg, and cheese as it contains 40 fat grams (fat equal to 10 pats of butter).

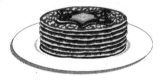

Hotcake platters are a better nutritional selection, especially if you don't pile them up with butter or margarine. They probably have less fat than scrambled egg platters. Burger King's French Toast Sticks have 622 calories— 150 calories more that Hardee's pancakes and more than triple the fat.

CHICKEN & FISH: Select baked or broiled fish or chicken breast without skin. Steer clear of chicken nuggets, BBQ chicken with skin, and deep-fried chicken or fish.

"Avoid fried onion rings, tater tots, or French fries."

DELI: Avoid high fat deli salads and choose plain salads and fruits instead. Choose lowfat sandwiches and bread or pitas with lowfat fillings. Limit cheese and meat to small portions.

DESSERTS: Select lowfat muffins, lowfat milk and shakes (limited basis), fruit salads, or frozen lowfat yogurt. Avoid chocolate chip cookies, danish, and fried pies.

FRIED FOODS: Avoid fried onion rings, tater tots, or French fries.

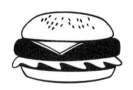

HAMBURGERS: Choose a medium or junior size burger and lowfat (e.g. McLean) when possible. Avoid adding bacon and cheese. You can pile on the lettuce and tomato or have a side salad with lemon juice or low-cal dressing.

PIZZA: Watch the pan pizza as it contains a lot of oil in the crust. Eat a modest serving of the reduced cheese variety. Vegetarian toppings are okay but limit the meat ones (e.g. sausage, hamburger, pepperoni). Stock up on extra salad and fruit.

ROAST BEEF: Lean roast beef without extra juices or cheese can be a lower fat selection than some other fast food alternatives.

GENERAL SUGGESTIONS:

"Omit cheese, mayonnaise, or top bun..."

- Ask for whole wheat buns.
- Choose whole roast potatoes, bean salads, corn, or peas.
- Drink ice tea, water, lowfat milk, or diet soft drink.
- Eat:
   —bran muffin without butter or margarine. Jam can be added for flavor.
   —broiled or roasted chicken and chicken sandwiches.
- Omit cheese, mayonnaise, or top bun on sandwiches.
- Remove:
   —crust from fish sandwiches.
   —skin and crust from fried chicken.
- Select:
   —lowfat regular and frozen yogurt.
   —pita bread stuffed with tuna or fresh vegetables.
- Try baked potato with salsa, low-calorie dressing, or plain yogurt.
- Use salad bars and limit dressing.

SPECIFIC SUGGESTIONS:

- Arby's: Try plain baked potato, lean beef, or roasted chicken breast.
- Carl Jrs.: Select California roast beef.
- Domino's: Order the cheese pizza.
- Hardee's: Eat one of their side salads.
- Jack-in-the-Box: Why not try the Club Pita?
- Wendy's: Try the chili or baked potato. Browse the salad bar and look for healthy choices.

BE AN INFORMED CONSUMER:

The following table gives some selected fast food breakfast items. It is arranged from low percent of calories from fat to high percent of calories from fat.

TABLE 20

ITEM	CALORIES	% FAT CALORIES	FAT (gms)	CHOLESTEROL (mg)	SODIUM (mg)
McDonald Apple Bran Muffin	190	0	0	0	230
Burger King Apple-Cinnamon Danish	390	30	13	19	305
McDonald Egg McMuffin	290	35	11	226	740
Burger King Bagel with egg and cheese	407	35	16	247	759
McDonald pancake with sausage	543	35	21	56	950
McDonald Apple Danish	390	41	18	25	370
Burger King Croissan'wich with egg and cheese	315	57	20	222	607

Exercise

This section is fairly lengthy since it deals with an area in which there is a lot of information *and* a lot of mis-information. For those that don't like to do a lot of reading, here's the capsule summary:

- Exercise may help preserve lean body mass during weight loss, but too much when on a low calorie weight reducing program can *further reduce* resting metabolic rate (which affects calories you burn). In fact, exercise increases short-term weight losses only minimally, if at all.
- Contrary to what was believed in the past, shorter but multiple exercise sessions may have the same benefit (at least for weight maintenance) as a single, long duration exercise session. Modest increases in activities of daily living have been shown to have greater long-term benefit to weight control than traditional aerobic programs.
- The most frequently recommended exercise by some weight reduction specialists is *gentle exercise* (e.g. walking). Exercise does not have to be punishing to be of benefit.
- Increased physical activity is possibly the single best factor in long-term weight control. Exercise has a very high correlation with preventing significant weight re-gain in people who start exercising during weight reduction or once they begin their weight maintenance phase.
- No matter what your genetic tendency, you should be able to lower your percentage of body fat if you eat less fat and do more continuous exercise.

DECREASED ACTIVITY & OBESITY

Being an inactive *couch potato* can be hazardous to your health. Television and other forms of inactivity are potent contributors to obesity. Many children and adults watch over 20 hours of TV per week and indulge in high calorie snacks while doing so. A study of over 6,000 men found that guys who watch more than three hours of TV a day are *twice as likely* to be overweight as those who watch less than an hour a day. Why do we join health clubs and then complain when we can't find the remote control for the TV? The secret of success with exercise is *regularity*. Limit TV viewing and plan healthy physical activities. If you are a parent, it is especially important to be an example to your children.

"...a multitude of physical and psychological barriers..."

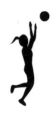

BARRIERS TO EXERCISE FOR THE OBESE

There may be a multitude of physical and psychological barriers which keep obese individuals from exercising. Several of the *physical* ones are a poor fitness level, as well as the added burden of the excess weight itself on joints and physical stamina.

Even more numerous may be *psychological* reasons impeding exercise. These can stem from previous negative experiences such as being teased, picked last for teams, or feelings of inadequacy. Someone may also be ashamed to be seen 'exercising in public' or may just not have the confidence to follow through with this important aspect of a healthier lifestyle. Try to counter such feelings by hanging some motivational posters (that you believe in) near your exercise equipment.

OBESITY & CALORIC EXPENDITURE

Some people who are obese may eat, as well as burn, the same or fewer calories than those who are normal weight. However, a number of physiologists think the obese burn more calories since they have a larger body mass to move around (hence more lean mass) but studies attempting to prove this have been conflicting .

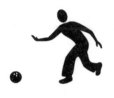

It may require several months for an inactive, overweight individual to become fit enough to exercise at a level that burns any meaningful amount of calories. Although the effects are not large, most studies find exercise promotes weight loss. Exercise has too frequently been looked upon as a new religion that glorifies muscles and sweat. A more rational approach is to be more relaxed and casual. Remove the *performance anxiety* that keeps many from starting or continuing with exercise. Realize that it isn't even necessary to lose weight in order to achieve some of the benefits of exercise. Results take time. Try not to get impatient with yourself.

ADJUNCT

"The cumulative effects...may be beneficial long term."

It is important to realize that exercise should be used as an adjunct (supplement) to your weight management program. Don't use it to justify eating additional calories. Since aging and inactivity are associated, a natural assumption would be that increased levels of activity would reduce body fat. However, exercise was not designed to lose massive amounts of weight and should not be used solely for this purpose. The Vasaloppet, an extremely tough 49-mile cross-country ski race in Sweden which lasts about 10 hours, requires the energy equivalent of only 2 pounds of fat.

The cumulative effects of even small increases in activity and exercise are what may be beneficial long term. Just taking two flights of stairs up and down daily, instead of the elevator, might provide 6 pounds of weight loss a year to an average man.

As a treatment for obesity, *exercise without dietary restriction* is not consistently effective. Any weight loss tends to be slight, if at all. Even with dieting, the average loss from exercise is about 4 to 7 pounds over and above any weight lost through dieting. Some benefit can be seen depending upon the duration of the exercise program. Utilized as part of a weight management program, exercise has many benefits, such as keeping the body's metabolic rate at a good level (increased calorie utilization), improving circulation, toning muscles, and strengthening the heart, lungs and musculoskeletal system.

> **FICTION:** Good amounts of weight loss can be achieved with exercise alone.
> **FACT:** Even though exercise increases the body's consumption of calories, it takes a lot of exercise to achieve weight loss without some sort of dietary restriction as part of the overall program.

"Sedentary living... important contributor to death..."

RISKS OF NOT BEING FIT

The time has come to recognize that low levels of activity and fitness are major risk factors for coronary heart disease and mortality from all causes. The results are in and the data no longer justifies the casual attitude toward physical activity that we have, even for those considered *healthy*. Sedentary living habits are an important contributor to death from coronary heart disease.

In studies on fitness and death, rates of heart disease are *seven to eight times higher* in unfit men and women than in those that are fit. Even the risk rates in other known unhealthy conditions (such as smoking, obesity, and hypercholesterolemia) are higher in those who are less fit and less active.

AGE RELATED FAT INCREASE

Activity and exercise has been recommended as a way for obese people to lower their percentage of body fat. It is known that body fat stores are increased with an increasingly sedentary lifestyle. An increase in percent body fat related to aging is believed to occur for several reasons. One of the current theories is that our energy intake (food; calories) doesn't always decline to match our declining energy needs as we get older. Another theory is that our basal metabolism falls, as does our activity level, as we age. In actuality, it is probably a combination of factors that influences this process.

EFFECTS OF EXERCISE

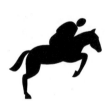

The thermic effects (increased calorie burning) from exercise have been clearly demonstrated, but the effects of exercise on basal metabolism are less clear. In the past, we used to think exercise always increased our body's resting metabolic rate, but some studies show no effect while others show some increase. Phinney, et.al. (1988) showed that exercise, when used with a low calorie diet, caused a greater *decrease* in resting metabolic rate than just a low calorie diet alone. The long term effects of this on weight loss are not known.

Since the functional capacity of the very obese may be so low, the actual amount of exercise that can be performed may be very small. Therefore, the overall energy expenditure from exercise may be fairly small in moderately and very obese persons.

"...exercise when it accommodates your schedule."

There is also controversy as to whether exercising at one time of day rather than another is better at burning fat. Some like to recommend exercising vigorously before mealtime as they feel this helps diminish appetite and helps control intake at meals. Also, since pre-meal vigorous exercise tends to reduce glycogen stores, incoming carbohydrates from ingested food may tend to replace these instead of being shunted to fat production. Since there has been no overwhelming consensus, prudent advice would be to exercise when it accommodates your schedule. One study found that 75% of morning exercisers were still exercising one year later compared to 50% of midday and 25% of evening exercisers.

"...don't exercise to get back at yourself."

ATTITUDE

Sometimes overweight individuals have a negative attitude about exercise because they are self-conscious about their bodies. This is just one of many barriers that has to be broken down to be successful in weight management and lifestyle change.

It's understandable why so many adults dislike exercise. Just think back to when you were in middle school and high school. Many times exercise was used as a *punishment*. How many times did you have to run laps or do push-ups because you dropped the ball or something not to the coach's liking? Too many of us still *punish ourselves* for over-eating through excessive exercise— "I have to go running *because* I ate too many French fries or a piece of cheesecake."

Get rid of that *punishment* aspect of exercise and concentrate on the fun part. Have a positive attitude and don't exercise to get back at yourself. Exercise is a neat and wonderful experience you can give your body and should be regarded that way. Let exercise be part of making yourself the very best you can be, rather than being a punishment for *being bad*. Add music and you may add enjoyment *and* endurance.

EXAMPLE SETTING

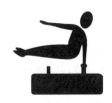

One positive impact you can have on your children is to introduce them to exercise at an early age. This doesn't mean just enrolling them in a kids aerobic class but by making them aware of your exercise program and what you do to keep fit. When you set a positive example by eating properly and staying active, you show your children a healthy lifestyle by example (the best kind of training). They will then be more apt to adopt your healthy habits as they grow into adulthood. You have a unique opportunity to influence your children while they are still young. Why not try to be a positive example for their sake and their future (and yours)?

"...health conditions and requirements vary..."

BENEFITS OF EXERCISE

While not all people will experience all the benefits listed below, and certainly there are other benefits not listed, the following list gives an overview (and hopefully gives encouragement to begin an activity program). Since individual health conditions and requirements vary, *consult your family physician* for recommendations as to the type and duration of any exercise program *before* beginning one.

Some Benefits of Exercise

Overall Benefits:
- Better psychological outlook (confidence, self-esteem)
- Burns calories (aerobic exercise burns fat)
- Can help arthritics move around more easily

- Could motivate smokers to quit smoking
- Energy increase
- Fewer GI disorders, promotes regularity and reduces constipation
- Improves general health and well-being

- Increases lean body mass
- Lowers stress and tension; can even reduce depression in some people
- May protect body against injury and disease
- Moderate amounts can decrease appetite
- Preserves mental abilities as we age
- Prevent middle-age spread
- Promotes better posture
- Reduced risk of sex hormone-sensitive cancers
- Sleeping habits may improve
- There is an inverse relationship between fitness level (exercise) and disease and death in overweight men and women

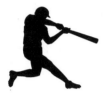

"Exercise... increases oxygen and nutrients in the blood..."

Nervous System:
- Increases oxygen and nutrients in the blood for better brain potential
- Stimulates brain areas that increase heart rate

Cardiac System
- Heart muscle grows stronger and pumps a greater volume of blood to the body
- Promotes a healthy heart and reduces risk of developing heart disease

Liver
- Helps control cholesterol
- Lowers triglycerides (lipids)
- Raises the level of high density lipoproteins (good-HDL-cholesterol)

Waistline
- Aids to decrease percent body fat which may decrease waistline
- Better weight maintenance after losing with exercise
- Physically active men and women have lower (more favorable) waist-to-hip ratios

"Helps control diabetes."

Muscles
- Increases blood circulation to muscles
- Increases muscle mass and efficiency (lean to fat ratio)
- Increases strength, balance, coordination, flexibility, speed, and endurance (especially in dynamic high intensity strength training)

Endocrine
- Helps control diabetes
- Lowers rate of developing non-insulin dependent diabetes (NIDDM)
- *May* increase some people's metabolic rate (though some studies are conflicting)

Respiratory System
- Increases depth of breathing and lung vital capacity
- Strengthens chest muscles

Circulation
- Blood capillaries in muscle enlarge
- Increase elasticity of the arteries
- Lowers blood pressure

Kidneys
- Effects blood flow
- Promotes output of hormones

Bones
- May decrease the degree of developing osteoporosis (if regular, weight-bearing activity)
- Improves joint motion

Tendons
- Improves range of motion
- Increases elasticity, helping the body be more limber

PRESERVING LEAN BODY MASS

One of the easiest fuels for our bodies to burn is protein, not fat. Since we want our bodies to burn the fat, we can use exercise (usually requiring weights) to protect the lean body mass and force the body to burn fat. One study showed that dieting women using exercise machines and weights lost about 85 percent of the weight as fat, in contrast to walkers and nonexercisers who lost only about 72 percent as fat.

Dieting alone can result in loss of both muscle tissue (lean body mass), fat tissue, and water. Exercise-only weight loss comes mainly from fats. Pavlou, et.al. (1985, 1989) examined body composition as a result of diet alone and by diet plus exercise in a group of people aged 26-52 who averaged 22% above ideal body weight. In the *diet only group*, the average weight lost was 5.3 kg of fat and 0.64 kg protein. Those who were in the *exercise group* lost 10.1 kg of fat and 0.11 kg of protein. This study shows that *exercise during weight loss* may help to preserve lean body mass.

"The easiest fuel for our bodies to burn is protein..."

As mentioned in an earlier section, exercise alone with no dietary restriction *may not be sufficient* to lose significant amounts of weight. However, in young and middle-aged athletes body fat stores are directly related to the amount of time spent exercising.

Exercise in combination with dietary restriction will not only improve fatty tissue loss but can also help in body re-proportioning by firming and toning muscles. When starting or increasing an exercise program, you need to be aware that when fat is lost and muscle is gained, there may be little change in *weight*. Yet, overall body fat has been reduced as seen by clothing fitting more loosely, even at a similar weight. This weight from improved muscles is okay since muscle is metabolically active. This means by developing your muscles through aerobic exercise and weight training, you can burn calories and fat much faster. It's the surplus fat that is the risk.

MUSCLE TONE

"...surplus fat that is the risk."

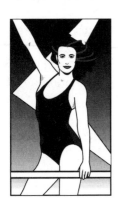

Despite the miracle promises of some advertisements, it is not possible to vibrate, roll, massage, or pound away fat from any particular part of the body. Body proportions are *entirely determined* by exercise's effect on underlying muscles (muscle tone) and total body fat and distribution.

You can help flatten your protruding abdomen by strengthening the abdominal wall muscles with active exercise of those muscle groups. Leg-raising and sit-ups are prime choices to help reduce the infamous *pot-belly*. As the abdominal muscles gain strength and become firmer, your stomach looks flatter and you look slimmer.

The following exercises can be performed in private, any time, at home or office with no special equipment necessary:

1) **Sit-ups**—Begin by lying on your back, with arms extended next to your head and legs together and straight. You may anchor your feet or toes under a piece of furniture (e.g. chair) to assist you. Bring your arms

forward above you and curl forward to a sitting position as you slide your hands along your legs and reach your ankles. Repeat.

A *modified version* for those with back problems (or just prefer to use it) starts with you lying down with legs together but bent (i.e. feet close to hips). Your arms are folded across your chest. Partially curl up, just enough to feel a strain on your abdomen, and hold that position briefly, then relax back down. Repeat.

2) **Leg-raise**—Begin by lying on your back, arms down by your side. With the legs straight (knees not bent), raise your feet 3 to 6 inches off the floor and hold them there for at least 4 seconds. Repeat.

You should do a few of these daily, probably before dressing in the morning as you will have less clothing to restrict your movements. If you are just starting with exercise, don't worry if you can only do one of each the first few times. You will eventually be able to increase the number as you continue your weight management program and work towards a healthier lifestyle. Set a goal of five to ten of these exercises every morning.

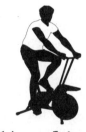

"*Aerobic exercise is not necessarily needed for weight loss...*"

AEROBIC EXERCISE

One way to *burn fat* is through aerobic (oxygen-using) exercise. Usual guidelines are that aerobic activity should be performed three to five times a week and last at least 35-45 minutes each session. NOTE: Aerobic exercise is not necessarily needed for weight loss, nor is it specifically recommended in obese individuals (*gentle exercise* is). *Consult your family physician* before undertaking any rigorous exercise program.

The Council on Fitness recommends a minimum of 20 minutes of a continual activity (plus a 5 minute warm-up and 5 minute cool-down) at least three times a week to obtain cardiovascular and respiratory benefits. The American College of Sports Medicine suggests exercising large muscle groups continually for 35-60 minutes three to five times a week to benefit your cardiovascular system. Walking, bicycling, dancing, swimming and jogging are good choices.

Aerobic activity sets a *target heart rate* to maintain throughout the activity. The target zone is determined by your age and fitness level, but usually ranges about 60 to 80 percent of your maximum heart rate, which is approximately 220 minus your age (as heartbeats per minute). The *talk-sing* test is a rough guide to whether you are in your target range or not. You *probably are* if you can carry on a conversation but can't sing.

If your primary goal is *just fitness* and not necessarily burning fat, then twenty minutes three times weekly should suffice. However, if fat burning is what you desire, then at least thirty-five minutes of exercise in your target heart range are

"...weight training does build muscle mass..."

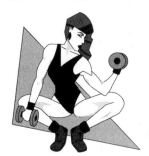

needed. Supposedly, the first fifteen to twenty minutes of aerobic activity uses energy from glucose or simple sugar. It isn't until at least fifteen minutes or so (*some say thirty minutes*) until the fats become mobilized to burn as calories.

Certain types of dancing can give you aerobic benefit—the Viennese waltz, rumba, tango, polka, cha-cha, samba, and the jitterbug. Square dancers get exercise benefit too as they may cover as much as 5 miles in a single night.

Even considering health limitations in some individuals, aerobic exercise is not for everybody. Such high-intensity exercise can increase anxiety, fatigue, and tension in some people.

ANAEROBIC ACTIVITY

Anaerobic (without oxygen) exercise is sometimes confused with aerobic exercise (mentioned above). During this form of exercise, your body burns carbohydrates and glucose (a simple sugar) for fuel. It is usually a start-stop activity like tennis, bowling, or weight training. Of note is that weight training does build muscle mass which ultimately assists in burning calories and fat at a higher rate when you do engage in aerobic activities.

WATER AEROBICS

For those people that are moderately or severely overweight, water aerobics gives a *good alternative* to the typical fast paced aerobics class. The water helps to keep you cool but provides buoyancy and resistance during the activities. Water supports 90% of your body weight, which is especially important if you have any musculoskeletal problem that limits jumping and bouncing. Aquatic exercise is *virtually no-impact* and so is safe for many people (check with your physician). Because water has 12 times more resistance than air, one hour of water exercise can be equivalent to two to three hours on land.

EXERCISE RECOMMENDATIONS

Not only do most weight reduction programs include exercise, but it is also recommended by many health authorities. To be effective in weight reduction, exercise should be:
- not too complicated
- performed at the same time each day (establish a pattern)
- a type approved by your physician (within your physical capacity)
- available without too much trouble or setbacks from bad weather
- focused primarily on developing a consistent (regular) form of activity

"...exercise should be part of a daily routine..."

Consult your personal physician *before* starting an exercise program, not after. Your doctor will be one of your best sources of information regarding *how much* and *what kind* of activity is right for you. Eliminate whatever risk factors you can before beginning. This includes reducing stress, stopping smoking, and losing excess body weight.

If you have risk factors and are less than 30 years old -or- if you are over 30 years of age and plan to get involved in fairly strenuous activity, have your doctor perform a stress test (treadmill electrocardiogram) before your exercise program. He or she may or may not feel that this is an absolute necessity, but it is well worth the piece of mind and reassurance it can provide.

Adequate fluid (water) intake is essential when participating in moderate activity to guard against heat prostration or dehydration. Drink water before, during and after exercise. Salt tablets are rarely needed in someone who maintains a healthy diet and generally should be avoided. Consult your doctor for further information regarding this.

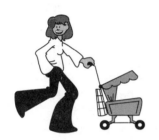

Proper clothing is essential. It should allow your body to breathe and perspiration to evaporate easily. Beware vinyl or rubber *body suits* as these can cause a buildup of excessive heat or even death.

Do not start an activity program by overdoing it the first few times. This will tend to discourage you and can cause bodily injury. Place your exercise equipment in the coolest part of the house and consider a fan to evaporate perspiration. *Work up to your goal*, don't start out at it.

"Beginning exercise is the toughest step..."

Whatever activity you select should be *something you enjoy*. It's generally recommended to build rest days into your exercise program. Consistency and practice will improve your skill and promote your enjoyment from it. Try listening to appropriate music as your exercise. Beginning exercise is the toughest step and sticking with it is the next hurdle. The majority of people joining health clubs (up to 80%) stop using them within six to nine months!

Regular *gentle* or aerobic exercise *combined with* a lowfat dietary intake is a winning system. You should not be exhausted or hurt a lot after the exercise, otherwise you are overdoing it. If soreness persists for several days afterwards, you were too strenuous. Vigorous exercise after a meal may cause stomach distress due to shunting blood needed for digestion to the muscles. Gentle post-meal exercise, like walking, doesn't make extreme metabolic and circulatory demands and can aid in movement of food through the digestive tract. It may also increase the thermic effect of food (may raise the energy *cost* of digesting food, though not always).

Avoid injury by starting with a walking program or weight-supported exercise such as cycling or swimming. *Be sure to warm-up* with stretching and calisthenics before the main activity to reduce the risk of muscle and joint injury. Competitive or body contact sports are not recommended, at least to begin with and for weight management.

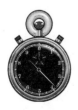

"Exercise longer, not harder!"

How much exercise is enough? If you desire to lose weight, to lose one pound a week requires about 500 calories a day deficit through eating, exercise, or both. An average exercise program for many people is about 30-45 minutes at a time. About the first 20 minutes of continuous exercise, you burn mostly sugar for energy. It takes a little longer to get to the fat. Exercise longer, not harder! Better fitness comes from *duration of exercise*, not over-exertion in a short time frame. The activity should be vigorous enough to cause heavy breathing, not leave you ready to call 9-1-1.

ACTIVITY OF DAILY LIVING (ADL)

Even though there are still proponents of aerobic and other types of exercise to promote weight loss and healthy bodies, many experts are now leaning towards recommending that people just increase their activities of daily living (ADL).

"...if you don't take care of yourself, who else will?"

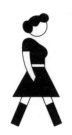

To accomplish this increased ADL, just look for opportunities to increase energy utilizing activities in your daily lifestyle, even if only for short periods throughout the course of a normal day. One study has shown that three 10-minute exercise sessions spread throughout the day can produce essentially the same fitness improvement as one 30-minute session. It has been found that it's the *total minutes of daily activity* rather than intensity or duration that is critical.

Long-term preservation of weight loss has a strong link with post-diet exercise habits. Studies show that among patients who lost weight and were able to keep it off several years after reducing, *a large majority* of them began exercising during weight reduction or shortly thereafter. The ultimate goal is to develop lifelong (not just temporary) exercise habits that help sustain weight maintenance. Even apart from its effects on weight, exercise reduces morbidity (disease) and mortality (death) even among the obese.

Keep moving as much *as possible all day* and do *just a little more* activity than you ordinarily do. Stand while talking on the telephone instead of sitting on the couch or at your desk. Take the stairs instead of the elevator. Park a little farther back from the front of the store or office so you have to walk a little further. Go an extra block or two to catch the bus or get off a block or two early coming home and walk the rest of the way (if possible and if you don't endanger yourself by doing this). Take your lunch to the park or another building to eat instead of at your desk.

Don't ride in the car for short distances. When on vacation, try walking more to sightsee and driving less. Depending upon your physical ability, walking may be a more suitable activity than jogging or swimming. It would be great if you could walk an extra mile a day, even if you feel you already do a lot of walking on your job.

Whatever activity you choose, avoid injury. This is why walking, low impact aerobics, or weight-supported exercise can be so appealing. You don't even have to do a lot to start with. Take a brisk walk at lunch or use the exercise bike while watching TV or listening to the radio. Why not begin with 10-20 minutes of something and progress to 30-45 minutes. Realize, this is *your time* and you are as important and special as anything else you do during the day. After all, if you don't take care of yourself, who else will?

"...walking ...can be ...gentle or vigorous..."

Since not everyone is a natural-born athlete, and since not everyone has the money or desire to join expensive private workout facilities or purchase special equipment, the ideal exercise almost suggests itself—walking! A key point to walking is that it can be *as gentle or vigorous* as it needs to be to fit individual limitations

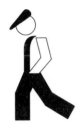

and can be an enjoyable daily habit. A slow pace can make it gentle while faster rates make it more vigorous. Even fast paces can be made tougher by altering the slope (grade) of the path—from a gradual slope to actually climbing stairs. If desired, it can even progress to running or jumping rope if physically fit. Realize that with walking you land with 1 to 1-1/2 times your body weight. Compare that to the 3 to 4 times body weight each stride supports with running.

Another key point for walking is that it is rarely impossible, unless the weather is really bad. Even then, many of us have shopping malls nearby or large, covered areas where we can go to get our daily dose of walking.

Walking tips:

"...walking ...is rarely impossible..."

- consume plenty of water and wear a hat in hot weather
- having a walking partner can sometimes be more motivational
- make time to walk (don't just try to *find it*) or do some other enjoyable physical activity *at least every other day*
- take 5-10 minutes to do gentle stretching exercise before the walk
- try to do something to burn 200-500 calories a day with exercise
- use appropriate clothing in hot, cold, or rainy weather
- walk with a comfortable long stride
- wear comfortable walking shoes (invest in a good pair)

Some might even consider purchasing treadmill type equipment or Nordic Track-type apparatus which allows them to walk inside the comfort and privacy of their homes. You don't even have to be so fancy as to buy the motor-driven belt treadmill, just look for one with an adjustable slope. A stationary bicycle is also okay if you can adjust pedal resistance.

Some people like to use swimming for a maintenance activity. However, others find that a moderate amount of swimming tends to *increase their appetite*, causing them to consume excessive calories. A brisk walk can accomplish the goal of exercising without the dramatic appetite increase that swimming can sometimes cause.

"What's the best exercise?"

> **FICTION:** More weight can be lost with a hard workout than can with a milder one.
> **FACT:** The exercise during a weight reduction program should be non-pressured, gradual, and relaxed. Vigorous exercise may cause more temporary fluid loss through heavy perspiration, which will be replaced later, but is probably no more effective long-term in true weight loss than a more conservative (but consistent) exercise regimen.

CROSS-TRAINING

Now for the ultimate question: "What's the best exercise?" The answer to that question is this, "The one that you will stay with the longest and be the most consistent with—hopefully for life!". A good recommendation is to *have several different physical activities* you participate in, perhaps a different one each day of the week. This way, you don't tend to get so bored or burned out on any one thing.

Aerobic activity can help increase bone density, relieve stress, and improve sleep habits. *Anaerobic activity* can be sociable, help reduce stress and tension, and can give different muscle groups a workout. Once again, variety is recommended.

GOALS

There can be many reasons for quitting a healthful exercise program. One main reason is that we select unrealistic goals to begin with. Instead of big and lofty goals, set many short-range goals for yourself. Take a realistic look at yourself, your present situation, your priorities, what you really expect from yourself, and then take the small steps first. This is where doing little things consistently, instead of big things inconsistently, pays off.

MAINTENANCE EXERCISE

"...establish an exercise habit that can be continued..."

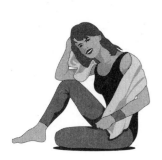

You should not begin maintenance activity until you have met the recommendations listed in this entire exercise section. Whatever you select for maintenance activity, whether increased activity of daily living, aerobic exercise, or a combination of the two, it *does not* take the place of proper eating habits, watching excess dietary fats, and healthy lifestyle habits. However, it should make it easier for you to maintain a desirable weight. As mentioned earlier, one of the *best long-term predictors* of weight maintenance was exercise that was *started or continued* during weight loss and *kept up* in the years after the weight reduction. Therefore, it's crucial to establish an exercise habit that can be continued long after calorie reduction ceases.

EQUIPMENT

Invest in the best equipment you can afford. If you can *try before you buy*, rent something to see if it's right for you. You might even want to improvise equipment, such as water-filled gallon plastic milk jugs for resistance work. Don't forget to check garage sales for used equipment. Many good intentioned people buy very expensive exercise equipment and use it only a few times before it ends up as a clothes rack.

"Purchase clothes that are comfortable..."

Purchase clothes that are comfortable and that don't restrict or inhibit your movements in any way. Get a good pair of walking shoes or running shoes depending upon your goals and preferences. You can't perform at your peak levels if you feel uncomfortable or don't feel good about yourself.

PROBLEMS USING EXERCISE TO LOSE WEIGHT

It has been determined that very-low-calorie diets combined with very vigorous exercise *may lower resting metabolism* an additional 4% or more *below* the usual 6% to 8% decline seen from the diet alone. Even with a slightly higher dietary intake of 800-900 calories, resting metabolism may fall when exercise is used with dieting.

Don't let this discourage you from exercising. Again, moderation seems to be the key. As mentioned previously, long-term maintenance of weight lost is usually better among those using very-low-calorie diets combined with exercise as opposed to those using diet alone.

PUTTING EXERCISE IN PERSPECTIVE

Physiologist Robert Neeves, Ph.D., has stated that one has to walk the entire length of a football field to burn off the calories contained in just *one* plain M & M candy. This may not seem like much until you realize it would require walking the length of the field about 55 times to burn the calories in just one small bagful (about 3.3 miles).

Certainly we don't have to exercise an equivalent amount for *every* calorie we eat, but we also cannot fool ourselves into thinking that a small amount of exercise will undo a lot of improper eating. If we don't walk the five hours and the equivalent of 240 football fields it takes to compensate for a shake, fries, and Big Mac, it doesn't take a genius to figure out what happens to the extra calories. Tighter fitting clothes usually give us a clue.

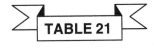

TABLE 21

CALORIC ACTIVITY CHART				
Average caloric expenditure for various activities - (10 MINUTES)				
LOCOMOTION	Body Weight (lbs)			
	125	150	175	200
Walking downstairs	56	67	78	88
Walking upstairs	146	175	202	229
Walking- 2 mph	29	35	40	46
Walking- 4 mph	52	62	72	81
Cycling-5.5 mph	42	50	58	67
HOUSEWORK				
Making beds	32	39	46	52
Washing windows	35	42	48	54
Dusting	22	27	31	35
Preparing a meal	32	39	46	52
Light gardening	30	36	42	47
Mowing grass (power)	34	41	47	53
House painting	29	35	40	46
RECREATION				
Badminton	43	52	65	75
Canoeing-4 mph	90	109	128	146
Dancing (moderate)	35	42	48	55
Golfing	33	40	48	55
Swimming (backstroke)	32	38	45	52

CAUSES OF FATIGUE

In dieters who exercise, undue fatigue is commonly caused by:

Inadequate food—particularly carbohydrates and foods high in iron and vitamins. If actively exercising, a level of *over* 1100 calories per day may help.

Inadequate water during exercise. Consume water before, during and after exercise, particularly in warm or hot weather. Dehydration saps your concentration and reduces your performance. It also allows lactic acid to accumulate in the muscle tissues, which can lead to easier fatigue and muscle pain.

"Consume water before, during and after exercise..."

Maintenance

Guidelines for managing your weight upon completion of this program are fairly simple. Even though the prospect of venturing out on your own may be frightening, you have learned most of the basic survival techniques and know many of the potential dietary and exercise traps and pitfalls that may lie along the way.

You may wish to go on *maintenance* for one of several reasons. You may have reached your goal weight and are *ready to graduate* from the weight reducing portion of this program, or perhaps you have *hit a plateau* in weight loss that is impeding your losing process. You may also be *bored* with your new lifestyle. The latter should not occur if you have undertaken small changes *gradually* and realize that this healthy eating program is not an *all or none* proposition. If needed, you can have an 'anything goes' hour once a week during which you eat anything you want. Many times, just knowing you have this set time for a splurge relieves the pressure healthy eating programs may place on you.

"...you have learned most of the basic survival techniques..."

If you are going on maintenance *due to not losing adequate weight* during the past month(s), do not be alarmed. Plateaus are physiologic and can be experienced by just about anyone. Do not be ashamed, scared, depressed, or have feelings of worthlessness, or even worse — failure! Just look on it as reaching an oasis or resting point. It can allow for psychological renewal and re-commitment (*mind-set is probably 90% of the battle*).

In general, tapering due to plateauing *or* finishing the program and reaching target weight is as follows:

1) Start to *increase* your caloric intake by fifty to a hundred calories *every few days* until you reach a maintenance caloric intake.
   - *This means that most women may go from an 800-1000 calorie per day intake to an eventual 1200-1400 calorie per day intake (and more). Men may start at perhaps 900-1200 calories and work up to around 1400-1600 calories daily (and more). These figures are arbitrary but do represent good ballpark figures as to where to begin once you have completed the weight reducing phase. If weight starts to be rapidly regained once off the program, these maintenance calories may need to be reduced slightly. However, it is not recommended to go below 1100 calories for any length of time unless you are utilizing the full program (calories, exercise, low fats, etc.) as you may reduce your body's metabolic rate.*

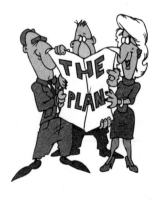

2) If weight remains stable or continues downward (if undesired), caloric intake can be gradually increased above the values given above. Physician or nutritionist input is advised. Eventually you should discover an optimum caloric intake to help maintain your desired weight.
3) In addition to maintenance calories, maintenance activity is crucial when off the program. Whether trying to maintain a specific weight

"Eat sensibly during the day..."

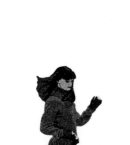

during a program oasis, or trying to keep additional weight off once goal weight is achieved, physical exercise (activity) is of paramount importance.

- *If exercise is something you shun or if the thought turns you off, think of it as being a stress reduction program, cardiovascular training, body shaping, or some other less repulsive term. All of these goals can be advanced with some regular form of aerobic exercise or increased activity of daily living. For further information regarding exercise, refer to the exercise section of this book.*

4) Maintenance exercise should be a minimum of three to four times a week within the guidelines stipulated in the exercise section (and within your physician's recommendations).

5) If weight starts to be gained, decrease daily calories slightly and increase exercise another twenty to thirty minutes. This should help you control your weight within three to four pounds monthly. The key is to perform these modifications when the weight gain is only a few pounds, not when it is ten pounds or more.

6) Plan ahead. If you know you are going out to eat Friday night and will be eating more calories than you normally would, Wednesday and Thursday cut back several hundred calories from your usual intake. This way, you *save up* some calories. Don't think you can overdo it Friday and then *pay it back* next week. Somehow those extra calories just never get re-paid (like our national debt).

- *Another tip is not to starve yourself all day if you will be 'partying' that night. Eat sensibly during the day so you won't be ravenous when you reach the banquet or party. Having a piece of fruit and a big glass of some low-calorie liquid before the occasion shouldn't hurt and it may help you make more sensible choices.*

In summary, weight maintenance is **maintenance calories** *plus* **maintenance activity**. One without the other just doesn't work nearly as well—especially long-term.

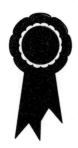

Congratulations! You have just demonstrated considerable will power and success in obtaining significant lifestyle changes. It is important not to fall back into a *comfort zone* and allow this weight to creep back on. Remember the analogy of being a *food-a-holic*. Like the alcoholic who has maintained sobriety for a few months you cannot afford to relax and just eat as you wish (watch frequencies and quantities of food). Now is the time you can really start enjoying your new figure, your new self esteem, and your new health.

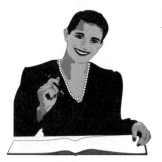

"Continue to have periodic, professional help."

How can you prevent backsliding? Please note the following recommendations:

1) Continue to have **periodic, professional help**. Experts know that maintaining weight loss can be even more difficult than losing the weight to begin with. For one year you will be at increased risk to start regaining, so it is recommended you have regular weight re-checks, at least every month, for the entire year.

2) **Exercise regularly**. Continue daily to look for ways to increase activity of daily living. Enjoy 20 minutes or more of gentle or aerobic exercises (walking, jogging, dancing, bicycling, etc.) daily.

3) **Commitment** is important. Select a reasonable weight range to maintain. Set a weight gain limit of 2-5 pounds over this range.

4) Continue periodic food intake notes (diary) looking mainly for trends and problem areas rather than absolutes. Continue **self-monitoring** for at least one year after you have reached your goal (longer is recommended). This includes the food and exercise journals, as well as occasional weigh-ins.

5) **Maintain fluid intake**. Consume 64-120 ounces of fluid daily. You should remember, many times thirst is misinterpreted as hunger.

6) Dietary recommendations:

   Avoid:
     —beef and pork more than 3 times a week.
     —fried foods and trim fat before cooking meat.
     —high fat luncheon meats, hot dogs, bologna, etc.
   Baked potatoes are OK as long as they are only lightly buttered.
   Eat:
     —2 to 4 servings of fruit daily.
     —3 to 5 vegetable servings, plus a salad daily.
     —at least 3 meals daily. Don't save all your food for one meal.
     —whole fruit in preference to fruit juice.
   Increase intake of fish and poultry.
   Less sodas, even diet sodas.
   Limit sweet treats or desserts to once a week.
   Read labels. Avoid hidden sugar, salt, and fats.
   Use:
     —butter or margarine sparingly, if at all.
     —lowfat milk.
     —unsweetened whole grain cereals, such as shredded wheat, Grape Nuts, Cheerios, All Bran and Nutri-Grain.
     —whole-grain bread and cereal products.

"Avoid hidden sugar, salt, and fats."

> **Myth:** It does not do any good to lose weight. You gain it all back sooner or later.
> **Correction:** It takes continued effort to keep the weight off, but the effort is well worthwhile, particularly if reversal of a disease process has taken place.

Long-Term Weight Control (1-5 years)

A. Maintaining Weight Loss

1) Treatment doesn't stop after weight loss (it should be on-going and life-long).
2) Individuals should continue with clinic or group attendance for at least one year.
3) Individuals should maintain support network (friends, groups) outside clinic or group.
4) The principal task is to learn to eat problem foods in a controlled fashion, as well as eating a variety of new lowfat, low calorie foods.

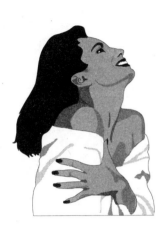

B. Preventing Relapse

1) Individuals must be prepared for inevitable lapses.
2) Clinic and helpmates must be prepared to intervene when multiple lapses lead to relapse and collapse.
3) Exercise program must be maintained to control body weight.
4) Changes in diet and behavior must be maintained to ensure healthy, balanced nutrition.
5) Weight-loss protocol should be resumed if participant regains five or more pounds.

The maintenance calorie level can vary considerably but is usually between 1300 to 2300 calories—depending upon age, gender, activity level, genetics, health status, etc. Maintenance becomes less frightening when your realize that your only have to have a decrease of 100 to 150 calories a day to lose and sustain a 10 to 15 pound weight loss (that's equivalent to 1/2 a Hershey bar).

"...be prepared for inevitable lapses"

Because obesity is a chronic problem requiring lifelong diligence in preventing relapse, it is recommended that individuals enter a maintenance program or at least maintain regular contact (one or two times per month) with their physician, support group, or weight counselor. Maintenance contact can be a phone call, individual visit, or group session led by a trained health professional.

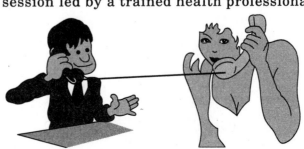

Children

The way you help heal the world is you start with your own family.—Mother Teresa.

Obesity is a common health problem in the United States. It is estimated that 25-30% of our children are obese. This is about a 60% increase in the past 20 years. About 20-25% of all teenagers are obese, which in itself is a 50% increase over the same time period. The sad part of these statistics is that 90-95% of these obese teenagers become obese adults.

Statistically, only about 1 in 30 obese teenagers will become a normal weight adult. All this occurs while in our world, forty thousand children starve to death every day. [Of course childhood obesity is only one risk factor for adult obesity since most obese adults were not obese children.]

"25-30% of our children are obese."

Start lowfat dietary habits early. There is a good chance if you or your spouse is overweight, so are your children. Eighty percent of children born to two obese parents, and about 40% of children born to one obese parent, become overweight. If both parents are thin, the chance of their child becoming obese drops to 7%.

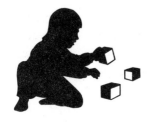

Weight after birth is not necessarily predictive of adult obesity but weight between 4 to 7 years of age does show considerable correlation. There is a strong suggestion that the *pre-school years are critical* in establishment of lifelong obesity in obese children. Body weight at age 7 has a high correlation with adult adiposity (fat). The weight at age 15 is a good predictor of whether the person will have an easy or hard time losing weight.

Begin your children on the right nutritional and exercise track from the start, and don't force them to make the same mistakes you have suffered through. Television watching, a major source of inactivity in children (as well as adults), is positively linked to obesity. Fat children are not cute, are not healthy, and do suffer from peer discrimination.

"Start lowfat dietary habits early."

Clinical treatment for childhood obesity should involve changing an inappropriate diet, providing an exercise program, and training parents about obesity, behavior modification, and associated subjects. Undertaking problem solving strategies as a family has shown better results than just individual therapy and counseling.

Have your child's height and weight checked regularly by a doctor and have them plot *weight for height* (instead of weight for age) to detect obesity. When plotted as stated, any weight-for-height over the 95 percentile is suspect.

The following is a listing of some of the problems that overweight children and teenagers may encounter:

- depression
- discrimination by peers and adults
- elevated lipids (cholesterol, triglycerides)
- hypertension
- irregular menstrual cycles
- negative body image
- poor self-esteem
- respiratory problems
- social isolation

Even though we are aware of the problem, we have to be careful not to be fanatical about the treatment of childhood obesity. Children need calories to grow normally and develop properly. Young children require a dietary intake of about 30% fat to help achieve proper growth and development. You can usually begin a lowfat diet for your children after they have reached age 2 to 3. Since half the calories in whole milk come from saturated fat, many authorities feel *children over the age of two* should drink only skim milk. They also require dietary intake of protein, fiber, grains, fruits, vegetables, vitamins and minerals—so low-calorie diets are usually *not recommended* for them.

The body mass index (BMI) of adults *adopted as children* showed no apparent effect from the family environment shared growing up with their adoptive parents. Yet, there was substantial biologic parent/offspring correlation. These and other studies have led to the conclusion that genetic influences largely determine whether a person *can* become obese, but it is the environment that governs whether the person *does* become obese, and to what extent.

"...average school lunch ...39% fat."

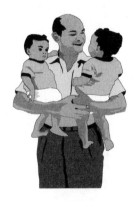

Looking at the fundamental problem on a national basis, we see that our children consume 40-50% of their total caloric intake as fat. The average school lunch gets 39 percent of its calories from fat. Therefore, any lowfat substitutions that can be made in their food preparation should be of benefit. Outside sources should supply the rest of their basic fat needs without parents contributing to the problem.

If we start to teach children about lowfat eating while they are young, they may not become adults with the same weight and cholesterol problems we have. Overweight children may need special assistance in learning to choose nutritious, lower fat diets, with adequate but not excessive calories. Encouraging physical activity individually and as a family can also be of benefit. The deepest and best lessons taught to our children come from *our examples*, not our advice.

The Center for Science in the Public Interest monitored Saturday morning TV food ads during the summer of 1991. *Ninety-six percent* of the food ads were for fatty fast foods, chips, sugary cereals, candy bars, and other nutritional catastrophes.

Clinical experience indicates that early childhood obesity is related to:

- genetic predisposition
- parental ignorance of the child's dietary and exercise needs
- parental difficulty in setting appropriate limits on undesirable behaviors

Generally, the sooner we help our children and pre-schoolers, the better the outcome. Several reasons mandate the benefit of early childhood intervention:

- it seems to be easier than in older children and teenagers
- parents have greater control over food when the child is younger
- less calories have to be saved to make a real difference
- may prevent chronicity (if fat cell numbers are kept lower, may be less of a problem as an adult)

Questions & Answers

Q. My cholesterol and/or triglycerides are high. How can I help to lower them?
A. Sometimes you can lower them just by losing weight. Other things that may be beneficial include reducing your cholesterol (remember eggs) and saturated fat intake (meats, dairy products). If you have elevations in these values, I recommend reducing your weight and then having the tests repeated. Don't forget that these values are more accurate after fasting for at least 12 to 18 hours.

Q. How much weight can I lose each month?
A. There are many variables that must be taken into consideration in answering such a question. It will depend upon how much weight you need to lose, your age, overall calorie intake, fat gram percentage, meal times, routine activity, other medications you may take from other physicians, and so forth. Several pounds lost weekly is considered a good amount of loss by many weight counselors. I prefer to have you concentrate on changing your *eating behavior* and *lifestyle* and the weight will generally take care of itself. However, if you concentrate on a certain *weight* and neglect needed changes in patterns and habits, then long term success is much more difficult.

"...take your measurements when you start..."

Q. Is it possible to lose *inches* without losing weight?
A. Yes. I recommend that you take your measurements when you start the program and recheck them from time to time. This will be an encouragement to you during those times where you might not feel you are making progress fast enough on the scale. However, if you slow down on pounds, you will eventually slow down on inch loss, so recheck your dietary intake and talk to your weight management counselor.

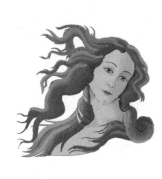

Q. Will I experience hair loss while on the program?
A. Some patients might notice this problem. However, it can occur in almost any patient who loses weight, whether on this program or not. It tends to be the body's nature to conserve during weight loss. Remember that hair is protein so be sure and get adequate protein while on this program. You may wish to obtain a *multiple amino acid supplement* (building blocks for proteins) from a pharmacy or health food store to take while on low caloric intake. If you do experience hair loss, you probably need to stay at the upper range of suggested calories. Either way, discuss this with your physician or weight counselor.

Q. I just can't seem to control my appetite. What should I do?
A. Review the suggestions in this book again. Watch your caffeine and/or alcohol intake, drink your suggested amount of fluid, don't forget your daily fruits, and greatly decrease your intake of food containing refined sugars and white flours. Eat more natural, whole grain items, vegetables, and fruits. Don't emphasize *dieting*—concentrate instead on eating properly and *changing* your previous behavior, especially in response to stress and boredom. Remember the *3 F's of Appetite Control*—**F**ruit, **F**luid, and **F**iber.

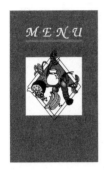

Q. Can I *spot reduce* fat on certain areas of my body?
A. Unfortunately, studies show that you have very little success trying to spot reduce selected areas of your body. Areas containing excess fat will usually shrink as you lose excess body weight. However, you can develop tone in selected body areas, which can give shape and firmness to compliment the appearance of these areas.

Q. Why doesn't this book list set menus to follow for the various low calorie goals you recommend?
A. I find that patient's food preferences are so varied that it would require a library of menus to meet everyone's likes and dislikes. If part of my menu included a cup of asparagus and you didn't like asparagus, then that menu would be wasted. As the old proverb goes, "Give a man a fish and you've fed him for a day. *Teach him to fish* and you've fed him for a lifetime!" This program is designed to teach you the basics so that you can fill in the framework with *your preferences and selections*. [If this book is being used as part of a weight reduction program, your counselor or physician may supply you with their recommendations or sample menus.]

Q. When is the best time to exercise?
A. There is no clear-cut consensus on this question. I just recommend for you to find whatever time of day that you can be the most *consistent*. Just look for ways to be more active *throughout the day*, even if it's only ten or fifteen minutes at a time. You might find it interesting that one study showed a greater number of morning exercisers maintained their exercise routine a year later than did midday or evening exercisers.

Q. I have trouble with chronic constipation and it seems to be aggravated when I try to lose weight. Any suggestions?
A. As you reduce your intake to reduce calories (and fats), your overall dietary bulk may tend to decrease. It is therefore important to concentrate on daily consumption of many *high fiber* items *and* adequate fluid intake. You should be aware that increasing bulk (fiber) intake *without* adequate fluid intake increase can actually aggravate constipation. You can also use Metamucil (try the low-calorie kind), FiberCon, or *Dieter's Tea*. This latter product can usually be found in a health food store and should be brewed *very weakly* the first several times it is used (try to limit use to only once or twice weekly if possible).

Q. Can *fasting* cleanse the body and help lose weight?
A. There is really no evidence that a *fast* cleanses your body's system of toxins or other unwanted substances. A self-imposed 24-hour fast for religious reasons or personal satisfaction is relatively safe for someone in good health. Fasting for longer than two or three days may be dangerous and is *not* considered a safe way to reduce excess weight. Total fasting for obesity leads to rapid fluid and mineral (electrolyte) loss rather than fat. Eventually you will lose some body fat, but you will also lose a lot of muscle (including heart muscle) and more essential minerals. It is definitely not worth the risks it imposes for temporary weight loss.

"...look for ways to be more active..."

Key Words

A

activity—increase activities of daily living (walking, stairs, etc.); make them part of your own lifetime program; find pleasurable ones (group and individual).

adequate—get proper amounts of proteins and carbohydrates in diet.

advance—prepare ahead of time for special events/situations; know alternatives and coping techniques.

alternatives—find substitutes for poor eating.

attitude—proper outlook can help or sabotage you; closely tied to expectations (make them realistic to improve attitude); perfectionism is impossible and *undesirable*.

automatic—avoid reflex eating and/or situations that cause it.

avoid—excess fats. This is the **#1** weight reduction tip! Also avoid the kitchen or eating *stimuli* whenever possible.

awareness—of calories and fats in foods; of eating. Food journals make this crystal clear. Behaviors cannot be changed until you realize you are doing them.

B

balance—in eating, physical, mental, and spiritual realms is to be sought after.

behavior—focus on this rather than actual weight; identify and break behavior links to inappropriate eating.

body fat—distribution of this has a very high correlation with many health risk factors.

C

calories—consider these instead of just the size and quantity of items eaten; weight reducers usually need to stay below 1,200 calories a day; weight *maintainers* range between 10 to 15 calories *times* their weight (e.g. 100 lbs—>1000-1500 cal/day). Low-calorie foods can be made appealing.

carbohydrates—increasing intake of complex carbohydrates helps many reducers with appetite and nutrients.

causes—obesity is rooted in many complex causes and interactions.

change—realize and get rid of unrealistic weight goals (e.g. fashion model/centerfold girls can range 12%-19% below ideal weights—some bordering on anorexia).

clean—plates do not have to be cleaned at the table to prevent starving children elsewhere, contrary to what mom may have told you.

consume—get most of your food/calorie consumption early in the day (e.g. by early afternoon); try not to eat after 8:00 p.m. if possible.

cravings—resist or learn to disregard these.

D

diary—self-monitoring of food intake and exercise with a diary is one of the few positive correlations with long-term weight management success.

dieting—avoid this concept because it implies short-term fixes, not long-term eating and lifestyle changes.

E

eating—do slowly and exclusively; enjoy each bite. Savor it like a true gourmet. Chew slower and more times per bite. Sit down while eating and only eat at one designated place.

exercise—many can benefit by just increasing calorie expenditure of things we already do (e.g. stand while talking on phone, take stairs instead of escalator, etc.). Find several enjoyable activities (both group and solo) and alternate to avoid boredom. Realize exercise is a *treat* and not a *punishment*.

F

fat—limit to no more than 30% of total calories in anyone over 2 years of age.

fiber—Americans need more of this in their diet; helps curb hunger; may reduce risk of certain cancers.

fitness—measured in many ways; pulse rate during and after exercise or stress is just one of many determinants used to evaluate this.

food—utilize the *new* basic four food groups; start minimizing food's prominence in your life.

fork—put it down between bites; pick up smaller quantities per bite.

G

goals—make them realistic; set long-term ones but concentrate on the short-term (daily) ones. Remember the story of the tortoise and the hare.

H

hunger—differentiate this from cravings.

hypoglycemia—this requires multiple smaller food intake throughout the day (at least an average of five daily). These smaller, but more frequent, meals may actually benefit other persons too.

I

incentives—non-food rewards can be utilized in a positive way to make behavior changes.

intake—reduce fat-containing foods; increase vegetables, fruits, grains, legumes; get adequate protein.

L

labels—read whenever possible, especially before buying or eating.

lapse—a temporary slip in behavior or eating desires. Catch and modify problem before it becomes a pattern (*relapse*).

leave—allow some food to remain on your plate. This shows you have control over food; get up from table when finished eating, especially if tempting foods remain in sight.

lifestyle—must be changed to be successful in healthy weight management. This is more important than temporary dieting and has been estimated to contribute over 50% to our health.

M

medication—may provide motivational assistance, nutritional supplementation and appetite training and should be physician-monitored.

must—a word to be eliminated from your vocabulary if realistic goals are to be obtained (e.g. "You *must* eat or not eat such and such" or "Exercise *must* be used to maintain weight lost"). Use *try to* or other such terms instead.

O

obsessed—if you feel controlled by food, get help. Contact Overeaters Anonymous, Take Off Pounds Sensibly (TOPS), or consult health care practitioners in your area.

omit—butter, margarine, high-calorie/high-fat sauces and other non-essential additives to typical American eating.

P

partner—a good friend or supportive spouse can help tremendously (tell them how). Eat, shop and exercise with them whenever possible.

patterns—discover these and ways to modify them (if inappropriate). Do this in your habits, your eating and your activities.

pause—take time to reflect: on life, your blessings, your goals. Do this during meals, throughout the day, at church or during times of high stress.

place—determine *one* (and only one) place where you will sit and eat meals, snacks, or anything. Stick to it!

plan—eating situations and meals. Make lists and decisions *ahead of time*, not spur of the moment.

portion—amounts eaten are very important. Try serving and eating *one* portion at a time.

preparation—meals and foods needing this generally allow for lowfat substitutions and can be healthier than fast-food or pre-packaged meals.

pressures—learn to cope with social and self-induced eating pressures. You have the *right* not to eat certain foodstuffs.

problems—daily coping and lifestyle difficulties can be discussed with your partner; health or medical problems should be discussed with your physician (the sooner, the better).

pyramid guide—visual representation of recommended quantity amounts of various food groups.

R

remove—take away serving dishes from the table. Remove *danger foods* from the home, car and office.

routine—beneficial in weight management if consistent, simple, and appropriate (eating, exercise, stress reduction, etc.).

S

schedule—may help you adapt to an appropriate routine. Try to eat as detailed elsewhere in this book.

shopping—do from a list and on a full stomach. Do it with a partner if necessary to prevent buying excess or unneeded items (or allow friend to grocery shop for you).

sight—'out of sight, out of mind' can be true with problem foods too. Hide them or place in opaque containers far back on shelves or in refrigerator.

situations—anticipate, plan, and recognize high-risk eating situations well in advance.

stairs—use whenever possible.

T

techniques—adapt and use lifestyle survival methods for eating away from home.

thinking—stop double-minded, out-moded dieting concepts.

triggers—recognize and modify situations, foods and moods that produce ineffective lifestyle responses, binges, or unhealthy eating.

U

urges—typically last twenty minutes or less for food; use diversion or willpower to outlast them.

V

variety—'the spice of life' and certainly true in good nutrition, exercise choices and behavior techniques.

vitamins—necessary in certain amounts for many of the body's needs. Variety in dietary intake will help supplement daily requirements.

W

walking—many Americans need to do more. Make it pleasurable (companion, radio, fun walks, etc.). Always warm up and cool down.

weigh—check weight at *reasonable* intervals (perhaps every four to seven days). Typically first morning weights in minimal clothing and after urinating are the best to follow. Warning: Do not be obsessed with the scale (a scale jockey)! Daily fluctuations are normal.

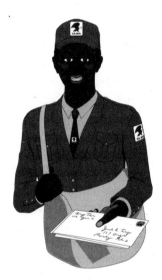

A Message From the Author—

If you get a chance, please drop me a line at the address on 'page ii' in the front of the book. I would be interested to know if this book was helpful to you or if you have suggestions, tips, lowfat recipes, etc. that might be helpful to others in a future edition. You may also write to me if you have questions regarding the spiritual aspect of 'total well-being' and I will be happy to send you additional material. God bless you and yours.
—Larry Richardson, M.D.

Index

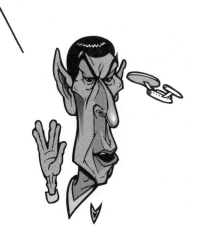

Captain,

There *does* seem to be intelligent life on this planet. The people reading this book are actually *eating* and *not dieting.*

Diets & Weight Loss

by Larry A. Richardson, M.D.

TO ORDER an extra copy of **Diets & Weight Loss**, complete this page and mail with payment (check or money order—no cash please) or credit card information to:

Larry A. Richardson, M.D.
ATTN: Order Dept.
2031 Humble Place Drive
Humble, Texas 77338

(Please PRINT or TYPE information)

Name_____

Address_____

City_____

State_____ Zip_____

Daytime Phone (_____)_____

Charge my:
VISA____ MasterCard____ American Express____

Acct. No._____ Exp. Date:_____

Signature_____

COST: $17.95 for book (Texas residents add 8.25% sales tax) + $3.00 postage & handling (U.S. addresses only). Check, money order, or credit card only.

Contact address above for information on quantity discounts.
Please allow 4 to 6 weeks for delivery.